Fifty Years Out
Physicians Reflect on Our Times

A collection of essays contributed by members of
the Harvard Medical School Class of 1953

Editors:
Fritz Loewenstein
A. Scott Earle
Donald N. Wysham

HOLLIS
PUBLISHING

ISBN-10: 1-884186-35-1
ISBN-13: 978-1-884186-35-6

Printed in the United States of America

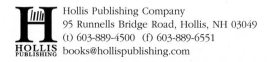

Hollis Publishing Company
95 Runnells Bridge Road, Hollis, NH 03049
(t) 603-889-4500 (f) 603-889-6551
HOLLIS PUBLISHING books@hollispublishing.com

Table of Contents

Medicine and the Law

Health, History, and Society

Miscellaneous Musings

Introduction

This book contains the views of a group of physicians about a variety of issues that have concerned them. The authors are graduates of the Harvard Medical School Class of 1953. Their views, recorded during 2003 and 2004, have been shaped by fifty years of experience as practitioners, surgeons, teachers, and researchers.

No attempt has been made to produce uniformity in the individual contributions to this volume. They vary in length, number of topics, and points of view. But they have in common dissatisfaction with shortcomings in our society, the state of health care, and the practice and teaching of medicine. Thus, these writings express the opinions, concerns, advice, and, we hope, wisdom, of a particular group of physicians on a large number of topics. The focus is primarily on health matters but also includes the environment, international affairs, national policies, and wars, all of which have an indirect effect on individual and public health.

Doctors are mortal. We have suffered the same diseases and incapacities as others, have become pill takers, and have had our share of joint replacement and coronary artery surgery. We have felt the emotional turmoil of those events and can better share the fears of our patients.

Unlike many of our patients, we have generally received good incomes and have had few personal financial difficulties. Yet we have learned from our patients of every background, rich and poor, their economic concerns, fears, and anxieties. We have learned that many have increasing financial problems, have lost good jobs, have difficulty making mortgage payments, are unable to afford expensive but necessary drugs, and feel vulnerable because of their inability to buy health insurance.

Some among us have been closely involved with environmental problems. Others have witnessed epidemics overseas or have been concerned with overpopulation resulting in lack of shelter, food, water, and sanitation. Another area of concern is the inefficient and ineffective method of handling medical malpractice cases. Nostalgia, apparent in some of the contributions to this book, may not always be justified. I would remind the reader that, until passage of the Medicare Act in 1965, many elderly people received no medical care at all.

We have witnessed a remarkable transition in medical science and practice during the second half of the twentieth century. As medical students in the early 1950s, we were still shown an occasional child with diphtheria. We saw tertiary syphilis in its various forms, and systemic uncontrollable tuberculosis (before the advent of AIDS). As a student at the Massachusetts General Hospital I saw leeches, obtained from a nearby Italian pharmacy, applied to the periorbital edema of a woman with thyroid overactivity. In the emergency room of Bellevue Hospital in New York City, where I worked as an intern, elderly men with deep leg wounds swarming with maggots were occasionally brought in from Lower East Side tenements.

Many of the contributors to this book have been agents in the technologic and social advances that have made such cases a part of history. However, as is emphasized in some of the following pages, the role of the compassionate physician has not— and must not—change.

All these matters, and others related to changes in health care and the medical profession, receive attention in this volume. The essays are intended for the general public as well as for health professionals. They may also interest those who contemplate a medical career.

I must emphasize that the writings presented here are the views of individual physicians. They do not represent policies or pronouncements of the Harvard Medical School.

Fritz Loewenstein
Binghamton, NY
July 2004

Medicine and Medical Education

~

What I Have Learned

Harvey Rothberg

Medical practice and the delivery of health care are continuing to evolve in our society. There is much that is new and much that is yet to be determined. But despite the ferment and the changes, the most essential aspects of medical practice and the doctor–patient relationship have not truly changed. They are eternal verities.

Like most of the physicians I know, I went into medicine with the altruistic notion of caring, of helping, and of being of service to others. Of course there were other appealing aspects of a medical career. These include the intellectual challenge of diagnosis and management of illness, the possibility of prevention of disease, the interactions with others involved in the health care enterprise, and the likelihood of achieving recognition and reward for my efforts.

When I retired from my practice, I was asked to say something to the medical staff of our hospital, "from someone who practiced for forty years without burnout and without a malpractice suit." I emphasized three things: (1) The unwritten contract between doctor and patient whereby the doctor is committed always to act to promote the welfare and well being of the patient. (2) The need for good communication between doctor and patient at every stage of their interaction. I sometimes think that communication is the most important aspect of internal medicine. (3) The limitations of medical intervention. We can cure some maladies, and sometimes effect healing and palliation; but there are also situations that are beyond our power to control.

American medicine in recent years has been marked by an increasing trend toward specialization and subspecialization. One of the newest specialists is the "hospitalist," a physician who confines his work to the care of patients during their stay in the hospital. The argument is that such specialists can manage hospital patients more efficiently and with greater precision in the delivery of expert care. This is particularly relevant for patients in intensive care units. The disadvantage of the hospitalist model is that the patient is cared for by a stranger who is unfamiliar with the patient's personal situation and past history, and unable to provide continuity of care after the hospital stay. So my personal instinct is to deplore the hospitalist movement, and to be happy that I practiced before this idea came to the fore. But I am aware there are studies which show that hospitalist care may shorten hospital stays by half a day or more, and thereby lead to a saving of costs.

An important aspect of the care of patients with terminal illness, whether it be cancer, neurologic disease, or a cardiac or pulmonary disorder, is the concept of hospice care. Hospice accepts the fact that cure is not always possible, and aggressive therapy may be or may become inappropriate. Instead, the emphasis is on palliative care, keeping the patient comfortable, controlling pain and anxiety, and providing fully for the spiritual and personal needs of the patient. There is no doubt that hospice nurses and other providers in hospice programs have enabled thousands of patients to live their final days with comfort and dignity, and that is good. But at the same time, I would hope that the primary doctor in such cases—or example, the oncologist whose chemotherapy is no longer effective—would continue to be involved in the care of his patient during the final period of his illness. Doctors need not, and should not, abandon patients just because they no longer have an effective remedy for their condition.

An important principle is specificity. This implies the necessity for individual decisions for individual patients and situations. Management decisions in health care, as in other aspects of human endeavor, must never be made in a stereotyped or routine manner, but always with regard to the particulars of the individual case.

Among the more frequently considered and emphasized concepts of ethical medical practice are the patient autonomy and the need for informed consent. Clearly, patients must have a central and active role in health care decisions, especially when there are alternative ways of dealing with particular situations. However, I feel strongly that physicians have a responsibility to provide guidance to their patients, who in many cases are necessarily naive with regard to understanding prognosis, and the implications—the potential risks as well as the potential benefits—of alternative courses of action. The challenge for the physician of course is to avoid an excess of paternalism.

Beyond Medicine: What I have learned over the years is not confined to medicine. Most notably, the fragile character of human life, and the unpredictability of the course of human events have impressed me. What happens is not pre-determined. And what individual humans do does matter. Men can change and shape events, if they will only make the effort.

A crucial aspect of a life well lived is personal integrity. It is important to do what is right, even when what one does is not popular or well received. Of course, different people have different philosophical or spiritual bases by which their behavior is guided. But if one is sure of the validity of his cause and his process, in the essential rightness of his thoughts and actions, he can live his life with confidence that he is on the right track.

Humility is an important concept, too often forgotten by some individuals. Despite the advances of science and the computer age, we do not know, we cannot know, everything. A corollary of this is that things are not always what they seem. And so I have learned not to believe everything that I hear, or everything that I read.

As regards the larger issues of the day, many of which have political implications: I deplore all forms of political or religious arrogance, as well as intransigent mindsets which lead to intolerance and to policies that fail to respect the rights and opinions of others.

I often reflect on the significance and influence of religious belief in western civilization. A mixed record. The Judeo–Christian tradition has been identified with high morality, grace, beneficence, and charity. But too often it has been marked by intolerance for other points of view, even leading to acts of cruelty and oppression. It is interesting and I think somewhat paradoxical that religious belief and observance continue to be far greater in the United States than in Europe, the continent from which most of our forbears came.

I deplore all those government policies that, influenced by pressure groups and financial supporters, allow environmental standards to deteriorate, permit too easy access to assault weapons, seek to prevent freedom of choice for women with unwanted pregnancies, and restrict dissemination of birth control information to people in over-populated and under-nourished third world countries.

Finally, I deplore the actions of an Administration that, in its zeal to remake the world, and on the basis of flawed perceptions and intelligence, conducted an essentially unilateral pre-emptive strike on Iraq, a distant and already degraded nation, without adequate planning and without regard for the consequences of its action. I have no doubt that the danger of terrorist actions against the United States and its citizens has increased as a result of the recklessness of an under-qualified and misguided president and his administration. Their policies have led to a decline in respect for America around the world, and an increase in hatred and contempt for America by many peoples. I suspect that if some of our leaders had been better students of history and of world civilization, and less involved with oil supply and with their sense of holy mission, these kinds of tragic errors would have been avoided.

We live in a complex and troubled world; there seems to be no end of insoluble problems. But we cannot give up the struggle. Despite the dangers of terrorism and the possibility of nuclear warfare, despite problems of over-population and environmental deterioration, there are still enough men and women of intelligence and good will around the world so that we can be hopeful that the future will be brighter for the inhabitants of this little planet. So I remain cautiously optimistic about what lies ahead.

Dr. Rothberg, a native of New Jersey, is a graduate of Princeton University and Harvard Medical School. He trained at the Massachusetts General Hospital and Walter Reed Army Institute of Research. For forty years, he was an internist and oncologist in the Princeton Medical Group. He is Clinical Professor of Medicine at Robert Wood Johnson School of Medicine. In retirement, he is a Docent at the Princeton University Art Museum.

Avarice and Health Care
Mathew Gelfand

The etiology of our present health care problem, greed, was first described 2500 years ago:

> *Beware an act of avarice; it is a bad and incurable disease.*
> —from The Maxims of Ptahhotpe,
> City Governor in Ancient Egypt, c. 2350 B.C.

And this disease has infected you, me, all of us, white people, people of color, Republicans and Democrats with equal frequency. Here follows a list of the symptoms of this condition:

1. A cardiologist gives an unnecessary five thousand dollar work-up because the HMO will pay for most of it with proper diagnostic coding.
2. Cosmetic surgeons' and dermatologists' fees for tummy tucks and other cosmetic procedures.
3. The overuse of MRIs, lab tests, by dishonest lawyers, chiropractors, and physicians.
4. Medications cost less to purchase outside of the United States.
5. A pharmaceutical company fined half a billion dollars for fraudulent advertising.
6. Cloning of medications. Do we really need all of the "statins," antihypertensive medications, etc., which are virtually identical in their actions and efficacy?
7. More pharmaceutical income is generated by treatment of erectile dysfunction than that of AIDS.
8. The concept that "everyone is entitled to the best medical care" is a myth. We have a multi-level health care hierarchy. The wealthy continue to get rapid and excessive attention. I know, for I have been forced to this route when caring for senators, members of congress, and corporate executives. Again, this disease infects Republicans and Democrats equally.

9. The high cost of maintaining Veterans' Administration hospitals, while neighboring mega-hospitals are merging because of excess beds.
10. Corporate executives indicted for fraud and corruption.

What is the cure for this illness? Look long into a mirror and observe that you and I are at fault, AND, *remember this on election day!*

———————

Dr. Gelfand remains active in the practice of internal medicine. He has served as Chief of Medicine at Long Beach Medical Center, and has been the Center's Director of the Methadone Maintenance Clinic for thirty five years. Dr. Gelfand was a pioneer in introducing thrombolytic reagents for the treatment of vascular disease (based on research carried out at Boston's Beth Israel Hospital), and methadone for treating opiate addiction. His nonprofessional interests include painting, classical music, and art collecting.

Compassion Governed by Common Sense
Edwin L. Carter

Growing up in the 1930s and '40s in a small West Virginia town along the Ohio River afforded me the pleasure of getting to know and talk in length with our family doctor to a degree few can enjoy today. As a lad who admired, respected, and honored physicians I considered Doc Harden my friend. Attracted to medicine at a young age, I soon recognized that he was the busiest of our community physicians. One day when we were chatting I wondered aloud as to how he had become so busy. He related that on arrival in Wellsburg from out of state he knew no one locally and opened a small office near the center of town. Initially he had no patients and he would come into the office in the morning and sit down to read. After a while he would go outside, saddle his horse, and ride lickety-split up through the town into the woods just north of the community. He would then stop and spend twenty to thirty minutes smoking his pipe, followed by a leisurely ride back through town to his office. After a suitable period of time he would head south and repeat the ritual, to be followed by a ride east again following the same script. The Ohio River was less than 100 yards to the west, precluding a ride in that direction.

It wasn't long before the townspeople began to talk about that new young doctor being so busy. It was only a short time before his riding had to be curtailed because of the rapidly growing number of patients. Was that marketing? In a way I suppose it was, subtle though it be. Doc Harden had a row of large, clear, glass jars on a shelf in his office, each jar containing pills of a different color. Each container's contents were identified with labels that listed the conditions that its contents were designed to treat, such as colds, food poisoning, sprained joints and so on. When he gave us a few of those pills from the appropriate jar we just knew we were going to be better. Only some

11

years later did I learn that no matter what the color of the pill, all of them were one-quarter grain phenobarbital. Doc Harden recognized, of course, that the vast majority of ailments that brought his patients to see him were self-limited and would resolve spontaneously. Some would call this quackery and deceit, but he listened, talked patiently, did his best to do no harm and worked magic in reassuring and comforting his patients. He knew the art of medicine. I do not recall ever hearing the word malpractice during those years. Today he would face charges of negligence or worse, but to us he was our friend, advisor and healer.

As a naive pre-medical student I had no perception of the radical changes medicine was to undergo in the next fifty years. Science was to unleash a plethora of advances in diagnosing and treating disease that few of us could have dreamed of as we entered medical school in the mid-twentieth century. All of us now benefit enormously from these extraordinary discoveries and innovations from the moment of birth and even before. As a society we have every reason to be grateful to the health sciences for these steady improvements in health care with a progressive lengthening of life span during this half-century.

Alas, during this time there has been a significant erosion of the perception of the universally revered and esteemed doctor of the first half of the century. For far too many Americans he has come to be viewed as a technician, a repairman, a medical provider, or a businessman. The evolution of the medical insurance industry with the encouragement of the Federal government has played a central role in this revolution of the manner in which the practicing physician is viewed. In many profound ways they have overseen major changes in the way medical care is rendered. Government agencies have urged second opinions, second-guessing, and have raised repeated doubts in the public's mind about the quality of care they have received from their physician. HMOs have repeatedly and routinely questioned the necessity of care, the quality of that care, and where it was to be provided. The steady drumbeat of doubting physician's judgment gradually, but progressively, has undermined the public's faith in physicians and hospitals.

Our medical institutions of higher learning have also contributed to these changes. Harvard Medical School fostered the development of one of the larger HMOs in New England with its subtle and not so subtle support of the Harvard Community Health Plan. Members of the Harvard School of Public Health were instrumental in the establishment of a fee schedule that was ultimately to become the basis for payment by federal and state governments and the private insurance industry to doctors and hospitals for their services.

The profound effects that third-party payers have had in eroding the physician–patient relationship cannot be overestimated. The physician has found his advice and decisions questioned at every turn. The insurance industry, the federal government, and consumer activists have striven to drive a wedge between patient and physician. Unfortunately, these efforts have been enormously successful.

Time is one of a physician's most valued assets, yet through a myriad of regulations third-party payers have sought to dictate our use of this crucial element of patient care. These rules and regulations have contributed mightily to the inability of the physician to spend the necessary time with his or her patient. These efforts by our government and health insurers to discredit physician care led to a rush of tort activities directed at all facets of health care. In the 1950s the judiciary began a process that in effect encouraged patients to sue. Activist judges pursued these activities in many areas of tort law, but they were especially active in medical malpractice in the 1960s and '70s. This resulted in a malpractice crisis that in turn engendered reforms in a number of states. This, in turn, brought a lull later in the 1970s in malpractice difficulties for physicians.

Within several years, however, problems resurfaced not only in the field of health care but across the broad spectrum of tort activity. Once again, a crisis prompted significant changes in tort litigation in the 1980s. Again, the changes were of the band-aid variety. Now the tort sickness has returned and involves the entire country. In the last few years there has been an increase in the frequency of claims, and even more important, a startling increase in the size of settlements and verdicts for plaintiffs. This has resulted in widespread physician dissatisfaction with loss of prestige and respect and a profession continuously on the defensive. The problems that some physicians are having in obtaining and paying for malpractice insurance is at or near crisis levels.

We have become a litigious society such as the world has never known. It is now generally recognized that tort activities consume 2.2 percent of our gross domestic product. Unless steps are taken to curtail such legal activities we can reasonably expect this number to continue to grow. The dollar amount is immense and represents a major liability to business activity throughout the country. Even worse, medical malpractice costs since 1975 have outpaced increases in overall tort costs, increasing at a rate of 11.9 percent per year.

The current malpractice system is an abject failure in its well-intentioned desires to compensate injured patients and promote safer medicine. Approximately sixty percent of every dollar spent in malpractice activities is absorbed by administrative costs, with legal fees being the major culprit. Rarely does a malpractice case move forward without the guidance of a trial lawyer with most plaintiffs' lawyers charging a contingency fee of about thirty five percent of any award. To compound the issue, only two percent of negligent injuries result in claims and only seventeen percent of claims appear to involve negligent injury. Thus, it is clear that we are dealing with a deeply flawed system for providing compensation to those truly injured by negligence. Ninety-eight out of one hundred patients do not sue when they are injured and five out of six who do sue do not have a meritorious case. It is equally clear there is a very limited connection between injury and litigation. The Harvard data from New York revealed that the degree of plaintiffs' disability rather than the presence of negligence was the overwhelming factor in plaintiffs' payment. We are mired in a system that is slow, steers too much money to trial lawyers, and fails to improve patient safety. The current system is a lottery where many plaintiffs' cases are lost when claims are made, but the skyrocketing size of jury awards that are made all too often to plaintiffs make trial lawyers very resistant to change. The average medical award has increased to one million dollars, a one hundred percent increase between 1997 and 2000.

In 2003 trial lawyers earned forty billion dollars from all tort activity in the United States. Tort litigation brought for medical malpractice in 2002 cost the economy as a whole nearly twenty five billion dollars. Is there any wonder trial lawyers fight tort reform at every turn? Yet studies have shown little or no relationship between payment of a claim and quality of care. Patients file litigation not infrequently over outcomes that no physician could reasonably be expected to prevent and far too many of these end up in court. Plaintiffs and their lawyers sue anyway, hoping they will hit the jackpot in awards for impossible-to-measure "pain and suffering." Jury trials with the present rules for expert witnesses have little or nothing to do with standards of care or getting at the truth.

Lawsuits are changing and complicating the lives of many physicians in ways that confound common sense. The filing of a malpractice action against a physician is often followed by years of uncertainty and bitterness, with the unlikely but possible risk of losing one's savings. There is widespread anguish in the medical profession with a feeling that malpractice litigation has gone beyond reasonable limits and that major reform is necessary. One suggested change is to establish tribunals to screen cases as is currently done in some states. In the states that now employ such a system the overall results have demonstrated a failure to weed out all but the most outrageous and frivolous suits, and in general have had no significant effect.

Caps on damage awards for non-economic issues such as pain and suffering are the most frequently considered and contentious reforms currently advocated by physicians. If this is to be meaningful it must be accompanied by a ban on waivers so as to prohibit runaway juries from circumventing the intent of such statutes. Other proposals include provisions to prevent plaintiffs from obtaining compensation for losses that can be recovered from other sources, particularly their health care insurer, in a procedure often referred to as double-dipping. Yet other proposals would limit lawyers' fees in malpractice litigation. These suggested changes represent a tinkering or revision of the current malpractice tort system. Politically this is probably the most the medical profession can hope to achieve at this time, given the large number of lawyers in the United States Senate and the pervasive influence wielded by trial lawyers in the Democratic party. Even limited reform legislation failed to pass in the Senate in 2003. Voting was largely along party lines, with forty-six Democrats and two Republicans voting "no" on a motion to bring medical liability reform legislation to the floor for debate. Medical liability reform faces an unknown future this year in the U.S. Senate.

Nevertheless, our political representatives are going to be forced to take some action in the near future to defuse this litigious time bomb. Unfortunately, we shall probably witness another band-aid approach to get us over the current crisis as politicians are wont to do, leaving the need for a completely new system unanswered.

I am troubled by the failure of our medical schools to participate actively in resolving this issue, one that is of overwhelming importance to the majority of their graduates. The public and its political representatives in Washington turn to these institutions for guidance and leadership in times of crisis. Unfortunately, our medical schools have for the most part remained silent, and this in effect condones and perpetuates the current system. I find this unacceptable and would urge others who feel likewise to make their unhappiness known to the leaders of their schools.

Our medical schools have a moral responsibility to contribute to and be actively engaged in the resolution of these issues. These schools cannot help but be aware of the unrelenting diminution of the public perception of physicians as a group and the loss of joy and satisfaction in the practice of medicine on the part of physicians. These truths will not for long be lost on would-be physicians contemplating a career in medicine. Our medical school leaders must rise to the challenge, discard the cloak of silence, and actively participate in our quest for a long-term solution. In contrast, we have witnessed efforts in some of the schools of public health to define the issues and possible means of resolution, especially at the Harvard School of Public Health.

Studdert, Mello, and Brennan have chronicled three avenues for consideration as a long-term solution (Health Policy Report Medical Malpractice New England J. Medicine, 2004; 350: 283–92):

1. Transfer of responsibility for patient injury from the individual physician to a health care institution such as a hospital or clinic, frequently referred to as an enterprise-liability model. This simply represents a shifting of the costs of patient injury from the doctor to an institution without addressing the issue of overall expenses of this tort action. It does not control the jury award system, and almost certainly the institutional entity would seek to recoup any costs from the physicians on staff. Furthermore, it is unclear how the individual family physician not associated with an institution would fit into this scheme. I do not see this as a viable long-term solution.
2. The so-called no-fault approach, which would establish a governmental administrative body somewhat akin to our

workers' compensation boards that would determine the amount of payment to be made for all medical injury claims. Such a body would award damages according to a set fee schedule. It is not at all clear this approach would reduce costs and in fact it is almost certain to engender an increased number of claims. This approach to the tort problem deserves additional investigation, but its promise seems limited.

3. Exploring other venues to resolve disputes is worthy of consideration. These include but are not limited to mediation, medical courts with personnel well versed in medical injury issues, and administrative law bodies that would be empowered to adjudicate such claims and award damages according to a payment fee schedule. Some have suggested these approaches be coupled with contracts signed in advance in which both parties agree to submit claims to the appropriate venue. This approach would seem to hold the most promise for a long-term resolution of the malpractice problem.

One small group of patients requires special consideration. This subset of patients, for a variety of reasons, involve circumstances that necessitate life-long support and care. If we assume that only seventeen percent of these cases involve negligence (the frequency determined of all claims filed that appear to have involved negligent care), we can conclude that over eighty percent of these individuals should receive no physician compensation. Society continues to wrestle with the issue of who should pay the millions of dollars necessary to care for these unfortunate patients. It does not make common sense to foist this responsibility solely on the physician when we know that quality of care bears little or no relation to payment of a claim. Many believe it is a burden to be borne by the public as a whole, for few individuals or families have the financial resources needed to provide the needed care. One possible solution would be for expenses for medical care and support above a certain arbitrary number, say five million dollars, be assumed by the government after necessity is determined by an appropriate administrative body. Under such a plan the physician would bear the responsibility for the initial five million dollars of costs.

A key feature of legislative reform must include thorough and careful investigation of physician misconduct. Every effort to disprove the myth that physicians simply ignore and hide inappropriate actions and errors of bad doctors must be encouraged. We must urge appropriate action against those who write improper prescriptions, trade sexual favors for drugs, administer care while impaired by alcohol or drugs, found guilty of fraud, as well as those convicted of a felony. A clear protocol for reporting each and every instance of patient injury must be established. It would be appropriate for regulation to begin at the institutional level with each patient injury or complaint being carefully evaluated by a panel of peers. If documentation confirms a breach of physician responsibility the panel would then make recommendations for appropriate action to the department chairman and the hospital director. Each investigation by the panel would be reported in detail to the state Board of Registration of Medicine, which could approve those recommendations or conduct an independent investigation if deemed necessary.

Another area worthy of review at the state and institutional levels is the issue of expert witnesses providing blatantly false testimony or distorting the truth. Disciplinary action must await those who deliberately lie. The problem of the "professional expert witness" is one that must be addressed. It is a fact that some such witnesses offer testimony in dozens of medical malpractice cases and earn hundreds of thousands of dollars from trial lawyers for their services. Misconduct on the part of these physicians in the form of lying under oath should call for disciplinary action and exclusion from subsequently appearing as an expert witness in malpractice actions.

These recommendations, if implemented, would appreciably increase the workload and responsibilities of the Board of Registration of Medicine in each state. Restoring the public's faith in the medical system is dependent upon adequate funding of these administrative bodies so that their mission can be accomplished. Whatever long-term program is finally legislated by the Federal government, it must preempt state statutes and be just to both the injured party and the physician. It is clear that physicians cannot continue to practice medicine under the current conditions. Without legislative relief the public is destined to see patient care and access increasingly jeopardized. The Massachusetts Board of Registration of Medicine reported in April 2003 that forty percent of neurosurgeons practicing in the commonwealth had paid a claim in the previous ten years. Thirty nine percent of obstetricians, twenty eight percent of orthopedists and twenty one percent of general surgeons had likewise paid a claim during that time. Claims filed, but no payment rendered, would obviously raise these numbers significantly. With jury awards now at the million-dollar average the current system is destined to collapse.

A physician is at risk of being sued with every patient encounter from morning to night, and if he or she answers the telephone at night the risk literally extends all day and night. Few Americans go to work each day worrying about whether they are going to be sued for some activity they perform that day, but many physicians do, especially in the high-risk specialties. Not only every patient but also every family member is a potential litigant. Once would-be neurosurgeons, obstetricians, surgeons and other high-risk specialists recognize the serious dangers posed by a tort system that is out of control there is no doubt that access to these vital services is going to be curtailed. It may take a few years but it will happen.

The malpractice mess is not insoluble. For the sake of both the injured patient and the physician a compassionate solution fair to both sides must be found. We can not go back to the days of Doc Harden, nor the golden years of the 1950s, but neither can we continue to go along with the current unjust system.

Dr. Carter was born in 1929 in Wellsburg, West Virginia. Upon completion of his surgical residency in 1960 he joined the surgical staff of the Massachusetts General Hospital. During his career he was appointed Assistant Clinical Professor of Surgery at Harvard Medical School. He retired from the active practice of surgery in 1998 and is currently an Honorary Surgeon at the Massachusetts General Hospital.

Three Essays

Harold Simon

I am a most fortunate man. My family and I emigrated as a unit to escape persecution in Nazi Germany and found a wonderful home in the United States. I was educated at some of this country's (and the world's) finest institutions of higher learning, thanks in part to the GI Bill, and under the tutelage of the finest teachers and role models. I entered the medical profession near the dawn of modern subspecialty medicine at a time when cures of hitherto lethal infections became possible. My colleagues and I were given the time, the opportunity, and the resources to pursue our professional development to the fullest extent possible and entered into our profession better prepared than any previous generation.

The advent of employer-sponsored medical insurance and, later, Medicare and Medicaid, made effective and affordable quality care available to large numbers of hitherto underserved persons.

Before our eyes medical science and technology devoted to prevention and treatment made giant strides that astonished and elated patients and physicians. The most highly qualified students sought a career in medicine. The future of medicine had never looked brighter.

In the more recent past, however, developments have thrown dark shadows over medical education and the financing of medical care. Further, improved and accelerated means of travel and the media's coverage of the human condition around the globe have served to inform us of the dismal conditions in which the majority of the world's population struggle to survive.

I will address three of these problems that I have been, and remain, deeply involved in both professionally and personally. These have intensified my feelings about my own good fortune and also shown me that the younger generation is generally much less fortunate, as is much of humanity around the world.

Disillusionment among Young Physicians

It is no secret that there is much unhappiness among physicians about managed care, reimbursements in the Medicare and Medicaid programs, malpractice litigation and insurance costs, the ever-present issues of the costs of medical care to be borne by patients, and other contemporary developments which adversely affect the practice of medicine. Articles in medical journals, the popular press and letters to the editors relate stories of physicians retiring early and suggest that, if they had it to do over again, they would not choose a medical career. Not so well known is another disturbing trend—an echo of these feelings among young physicians. Why is this happening?

Then: When we were medical students and house officers, the idea of abandoning a career in medicine was inconceivable. We had worked hard, overcome numerous obstacles, and eagerly looked ahead to a highly satisfying career helping to heal the sick. World War II had led to numerous medical advances; the age of antimicrobials had dawned and promised effective cures for hitherto often lethal infections, and demonstrated the effectiveness of specialized training and care.

In the undergraduate clinical years and during our residencies we were taught and supervised by highly skilled, broadly competent, and—for the most part—humanistically oriented clinicians and clinician-scientists who became our role models.

The financial aspects of patient care almost never intruded on our education as medical students or residents. So long as relevance to the matter at hand could be shown, if a question about a diagnosis arose, or in pursuit of a matter of clinical education, we were able to order the desired investigations without considering the costs.

Medicine became our vocation and avocation. We spent every day and at least every second night on service. A patient admitted to our care had usually been seen only by a referring physician or for triage in a clinic. Our continuous presence on service enabled us to obtain the medical history, perform physical examinations, order investigational steps, initiate therapy and observe the results of our interventions. We stayed with and followed our patients' progress.

We learned our profession from more senior residents, attending physicians, and broadly competent "compleat physician" chiefs of service who taught us how to approach a patient and his or her problems, avoid or rectify errors and mistakes, and communicate our questions, ideas and suggestions to colleagues, patients and their families.

Today: As a medical school professor with a long history as dean of admissions, student affairs and curriculum, I am too often confronted by a young resident who is seriously considering abandoning medicine for a different career. This, after more than a decade of study in college, participating in the grueling competition to enter medical school, a rigorous undergraduate medical education, passing the board examinations, and competing again for a prized residency position.

My observations as to the reasons for this deplorable situation lead me to point to the following factors:

On entering medical school, today's students are not much different from the highly intelligent, strongly motivated, largely idealistic young people of yesteryear. As undergraduate medical students, they are not sufficiently prepared for the current realities of medical practice as these differ from their idealistic expectations. As residents, they find that the differences include the continuous intrusion of financial factors affecting their efforts to study and care for their patients' problems. A part of their clinical practice tries to prevent potential malpractice litigation.

The "compleat physician" role models have been replaced for the most part by physicians more focused on their own subspecialized clinical topics and research than on broadly addressing patients' problems or students' needs. Moreover, many clinical teachers must devote a great deal of time to clinical practice in order to generate income for themselves and their home institution.

Today's residents on in-patient services are largely deprived of the excitement entailed in approaching a patient who has not already been extensively examined. Instead of establishing a differential diagnosis and a plan for further investigation, beginning treatment, and observing its effects, residents on hospital in-patient services see patients whose problems have often been identified before admission, who come in for a specific investigational or therapeutic procedure, and who leave the hospital well before the effects of treatment have become apparent.

23

The problem of limited follow-up as a consequence of short hospital stays is compounded by the fact that residents spend only every third or fourth night on service. On outpatient services, the need to rush patients along as a consequence of financial concerns and attending physicians' other commitments beyond teaching accentuates these problems.

At the same time, residents may be confronted for the first time by the realities of managed care, considerations of malpractice litigation, and—perhaps above all—by a great deal of negative counseling about the allegedly dismal state of medical practice in the United States today. They may have heard some of this before entering medical school but may not have paid attention until personally and directly confronted with some of these issues. Coming at a time when these young people are tired, feel stressed and overworked, it is perhaps no wonder that some become disenchanted and look for escape. In addition, most of today's medical students graduate deeply in debt, which affects career choice, location and mode of practice.

This situation is all the more deplorable because these feelings come at a time when the future of clinical medicine has never been brighter. Progress in biomedical research, both at basic and applied levels, promises a very bright future for diagnostic studies and therapeutic interventions.

What To Do? The problems identified above—the constraints on detailed investigation and observation of patients, the financial aspects of medical practice and medical care, the malpractice threat, the issues pertaining to role models, and the intrusion of managers' decision making in medical care—will undoubtedly persist, at least for the immediate future. Thus, we need to find means to address these issues in context of the larger issues of a career in medicine.

I believe I am addressing a problem among a minority of young physicians at present, but one that is growing. There is need to recognize and understand the reasons for the disillusionment among young physicians concerning a career in medicine. Some are cited above. I believe these must be addressed early and directly to young people contemplating a medical career. They need to be much better informed about both the very bright future of medicine in terms of meeting the preventive and therapeutic needs of patients and about those aspects of medical practice which may differ significantly from their romantic or idealistic expectations.

Career days, information in printed and electronic media, counseling provided by well-informed and dedicated physicians practicing in diverse communities, and by physician-scientists working to discover and apply biomedical advances for patient care need to be more prevalent and widely advertised.

The pre-clinical components of the medical school curriculum address the exciting promises and frontiers of biomedical science. However, the realities of medical practice are likely to be addressed much less effectively, and often not until the residency years, or even later. The need clearly exists to inform rising physicians quite early and continuously about both the positive and the negative aspects of clinical practice.

These matters are or should be of interest and concern at least to medical teachers, to the American, National and State Medical Associations, and to the Association of American Medical Colleges. Their efforts to address and inform rising physicians would doubtless prove useful and effective in stemming and perhaps reversing the rising disillusionment among those highly intelligent and motivated young people aiming at a medical career.

$\sim$

The Uninsured

Some 44 million Americans are uninsured for health care, and their numbers are rising. The great majority are employees of companies which do not offer employer-sponsored medical insurance. The United States, the leader of the "Free World" and its richest member, is the only industrialized country which does not provide essentially universal health insurance. The clear consequences of this apparent lack of concern for the less fortunate include greater use of emergency and critical care facilities for routine and advanced medical problems, neglect of preventive measures and reduced use of medical technology, including medicaments, all resulting in unnecessary misery and mortality and, eventually, unnecessarily greater costs to the health care delivery system.

The rising number of the uninsured and the consequences noted above were clearly foreseen long ago. In the early 1990s, the Clinton Administration attempted to address and ameliorate this situation. In fact, this period seemed to coincide with an opportunity appearing approximately once in every generation to effect significant changes and improvements in health care delivery in the United States. The effort failed, not least because it failed to include effective spokespersons for the principal stakeholders—hospitals, physicians, and insurance companies—and because the proposals which eventually emerged were perhaps too sweeping and all-encompassing to be addressed effectively in the requisite political process.

There can be little doubt that the issue of the uninsured is among *the* most pressing if not the most pressing problem confronting the provision of medical care in the United States today. In addition to the adverse health and medical consequences cited above, the more recently emerging concerns about usage of biologic and other weapons of mass destruction (and natural catastrophes such as Hurricane Katrina) raise the specter of a sudden massive need to treat large numbers of casualties whose health insurance status will most likely be in doubt.

And there are additional serious economic consequences, as well. For example, the American automobile industry indicates that the costs of every automobile produced here include more than $1,200 for workers' health insurance. By contrast, and thanks to universal health insurance, a Canadian automaker has no such costs and, despite higher taxes, realizes significant cost advantages in comparison to his American counterpart.

Then there is the much-lamented and increasing practice of outsourcing work, which causes losses of jobs at home. The reasons are easy to identify. They include lower labor costs overall. Usually, employer-paid health insurance is also not included in workers' compensation. These factors put economic pressures on employers at home for which outsourcing is at least a temporary remedy.

What To Do? I believe that the only potentially effective means to address these problems and the resultant adverse health and economic consequences reside in some form of universal health insurance. Time-proven American ingenuity and inventiveness should enable our experts and policy makers to study and learn from both the strengths and weaknesses of universal health care systems elsewhere. Also, policy makers should look to overcome the mistakes that were made in the course of the attempt to implement such a system in the early 1990s.

Such a system need not be government-run but government must clearly play an essential role in its formulation and implementation. Halfway or state by state measures cannot succeed, as shown by the example of Tennessee (although Hawaii's experiment seems to be succeeding—but that is a very special case). Undoubtedly, there would be massive savings in administrative time and costs if a universal system were adopted, some or most of which could go into the costs of providing care for the currently uninsured population.

This idea has numerous opponents who point to the flaws in extant universal health care delivery systems. But it also has a great many advocates among health policy experts and, most recently, from the Institute of Medicine.

For myself, I see no other way by which this enormous problem can be addressed effectively. And I believe it is high time for another attempt to solve the problems of the uninsured.

∽

International Health: Problems, Implications, Remedies

Where health and health care are concerned, the world is deeply divided into two camps—the fortunate and the unfortunate. The industrialized countries of North America, Western Europe, Japan, Australia and New Zealand (often referred to as "The North"—numbering roughly one fourth of the world's population—compose the former. Most of the rest of the world ("The South") must be counted among the latter. Mass travel and occasional reports in the media are gradually calling attention to the great differences in health status between these two worlds. Belatedly, some recent public and private initiatives have been forged to bridge the gaps between them.

In the industrialized countries, the principal causes of premature deaths are due to heart disease, cancer, stroke, interpersonal violence, and traffic accidents. Infectious diseases of major concern are represented almost exclusively by influenza, pneumonia, and HIV/AIDS. In the developing world, on the other hand, where these same chronic diseases and violence are becoming increasingly prevalent, a majority of premature deaths is due to infectious diseases. Effective prevention and treatments exist for most of these in the forms of environmental sanitation, immunizations, and antibiotics (see the table below). Such measures are not available to many people for a variety of reasons. At the individual level, these include poverty, lack of education about health matters, unhealthy traditional practices, and remoteness of domiciles. At the national level, inappropriate priorities and administrative decisions, inadequate infrastructure, lack of finances for public health efforts, and a focus on health care delivery in the capital and major cities with neglect of rural communities form a malignant constellation which fails to address major health and medical problems and leads to an unnecessarily heavy burden of illness and death.

Examples abound, as shown in the table below (numbers rounded):

Year 2000	Industrialized world	Developing world
World population: 6 billion	1.5 billion (25%)	4.5 billion (75%)
Annual deaths: 52 million	10 million (<20%)	42 million (>80%)
Deaths from infectious diseases: 17 million	<10%	>90%

The Developing World's Ten Biggest Killers (Deaths per annum)

Acute lower respiratory infections	4.4 million (90% children)
Diarrheal diseases**	3.1 million (95% children)
Tuberculosis*	3.1 million (mostly adults)
Malaria	2.1 million (50% children)
Hepatitis B*,**	1.1 million (mostly adults)
HIV/AIDS	1.1 million (rising steeply)
Measles*	1.0 million (children)
Neonatal tetanus*	1.0 million (infants)
Whooping cough*	0.5 million (infants, children)
Intestinal worms**	150,000

The Developing World's Ten Most Common Infectious Disease Problems

Diarrheal diseases**	4 billion episodes annually
Tuberculosis*	2 billion active cases
Intestinal worms**	2 billion active cases
Malaria	500 million new episodes annually
Hepatitis B*	350 million chronic carriers
Hepatitis C**	100 million active carriers
Acute lower respiratory infections	500 million episodes annually
Sexually transmitted diseases	400 million episodes annually
Measles*	45 million episodes annually
Whooping cough*	40 million episodes annually

*Vaccine preventable
**Safe water/sanitation preventable
Disease statistics from the World Health Organizaton

In addition, approximately 1 billion people are malnourished, of whom about 15% are children. Bad enough of and by itself, this tragedy's consequences among infants and children include stunted mental and physical growth and development, heightened susceptibility to a variety of infectious diseases and premature death, and impaired work performance throughout life. Among adults, malnutrition plays a major role in a life of impaired work performance and continuing poverty. In addition to inadequate protein and caloric intake, malnutrition usually entails insufficient intake of vitamins, minerals, and trace elements resulting in disease states specifically attributable to these deficiencies.

To continue with this litany of horrors, most people in the developing world live either in cities under conditions of squalor—overcrowded shanty towns that foster interpersonal violence and epidemics, environmental pollution, and absence of municipal services such as electric power and running water; or they live in rural settings, eking out a bare existence, and usually remote from effective health and medical services. They may be exposed to pesticides and other environmental pollutants, and are often subject to raids by armed bands of murderers and pillagers. There is generally no governmental protection against these conditions and abuses.

This is the fertile soil in which hopelessness and despair originate and thrive. With promises of a better life in the hereafter, demagogues and religious fanatics find easy pickings among the young, the desperate and the angry to undertake acts of violence and self-immolation directed against designated targets.

To add another malignant dimension: With few exceptions, medical education in The South generally attempts to emulate its counterparts in The North, and specifically the pattern set in the United States. The stress is on science-based and technologically oriented medical practice. Often, the best and the brightest pursue advanced training in the hospitals and research institutions of The North. Upon completion, these highly trained physicians face the prospect of a return to under equipped work sites and elect instead to become part of the "brain drain" by remaining in The North. A similar pattern is found in the education and training of scientists. Taken together, this deprives The South of potential leaders and innovators in their fields who will not be devoting their talents and energy to address the dire needs of the developing countries.

The North has made some efforts aimed at ameliorating the enormous gaps between conditions in the two worlds by means of bilateral projects and in support of the World Health Organization's (WHO) activities. Notable successes have been achieved in the past quarter century as exemplified by the eradication of smallpox and the imminent elimination of polio worldwide, and by major reductions in the prevalence of some parasitic infections in Africa and Asia, notably dracunculosis (dragontiasis) and river blindness (onchocerciasis).

But much remains to be done. In addition to the traditional scourges which have plagued the developing countries since time immemorial, new problems have arisen. First and foremost is the uncontrolled pandemic of HIV/AIDS which, in Africa, is fomenting an avalanche of orphans, a massive increase in tuberculosis, and devastation of political, economic and social fabrics. Although not yet apparent, a similar fate threatens the world's two most populous countries: India and the Peoples Republic of China.

Additional examples may be cited to demonstrate that the world—and not only The South—is under continuous threat to our health and well-being. Again, with a focus on infectious disease problems numerous illustrative examples may be cited. These include, among others:

- the resurgence of drug- and pesticide-resistant malaria;
- the sudden emergence of epizootic H5N1 avian influenza in Asia with its potential to engender a world-wide pandemic possibly even worse than the 1918–20 variety;
- the unexpected and novel appearance of SARS (serious acute respiratory syndrome) in East Asia and its almost immediate spread to North America;
- the reappearance of cholera in the Western Hemisphere after almost a full century's absence;
- the spread of dengue fever northward into the United States;
- the emergence and spread of a variety of highly lethal hemorrhagic virus infections from their previously remote habitats in the African jungle as a result of human encroachment; and
- the possibility that, in native or modified form, these may be made into weapons for bioterrorists.

In our troubled times, this last item deserves further emphasis. The threat of bioterrorism has highlighted the many inadequacies in the American public health system after more than a generation of neglect. As a partial response to a few recent cases of anthrax traced to deliberately contaminated mail, a significant amount of additional federal funding has been authorized toward improvement of the system. This effort is aimed particularly at development of technology for early and rapid detection of infectious agents potentially employed in acts of bioterrorism and their prevention and treatment. This may be appropriate as a relatively short-term approach. It will take much longer and may require fundamental changes in our educational system to address the critical shortages of trained public health public health personnel.

The United States is the only industrialized country in which education in matters pertaining to public health is almost completely separate from medical education. Thus, since medically trained personnel are likely to be among the first responders to a bioterrorism event, and early responses must rely heavily on public health measures to be effective, it is essential that medical education incorporate basic principles of public health measures, strategies and tactics. This applies not only to acts of bioterrorism but also to potential epidemics, such as influenza, or newly appearing problems, such as the recent emergence of SARS and H5N1 influenza. To date, there is little evidence that this need has been recognized, let alone addressed. Thus, whereas the health problems of The South clearly demand attention in their own right, it is (or should be) just as obvious that it is in The North's own interest to devote talent and treasure toward their control.

Efforts to address international health problems by means of foreign aid have indeed been undertaken by the industrial powers ever since the time of colonial imperialism. More recently, the Scandinavian countries and Canada in particular have allocated significant fractions of their resources to foreign aid, much of it in the form of bilateral projects devoted to development and improvement of infrastructure and education. Sad to say, the United States has devoted the smallest fraction of its resources for such purposes.

Recently, the United States has committed to increasing its contributions both directly and via the World Health Organization to address some specific health problems affecting The South (with echoes in The North), including HIV/AIDS, tuberculosis, and malaria. The United States may be said to be following the lead of the private sector, most notably the Gates Foundation, in finally recognizing the urgent need for such assistance. But much more is needed!

By now it should be obvious that we in The North forget or ignore The South's problems at our peril. Geopolitically, economically, in consideration of the depletion of natural resources, and with a view to ongoing environmental degradation, whatever happens in one part of the world must now be seen to have ramifications almost everywhere. It is high time for The North to recognize that this is indeed "One World." It is incumbent upon all of us to become better informed about the health and well-being—and the lack thereof—of all those with whom we share this small planet. For one part of the world's problems can no longer be limited to that part nor put out of mind. We are all in this together and are destined to sink or swim together.

After immigrating from Germany, Dr. Simon settled in San Francisco in 1939. Following medical school, he trained in internal medicine at the New York Hospital and thereafter received his Ph.D degree from Rockefeller University. He served on the medical faculty at Stanford and later became Dean of students and Professor of Family and Preventive Medicine at the University of California, San Diego. Dr. Simon established the Division of International Health and Cross-Cultural Medicine at the Institue of Medicine and subsequently at UCSD. Formally retired, he is still in full-time academic medicine.

Providing Health Care in the United States

Charles G. Barnett

The Problem of Increasing Health Care Costs: During the past several decades, the delivery of health care in the United States has become progressively more expensive, with increasing barriers to access for the average citizen. The heart of the problem is economic, and it is here that we should focus our attention. Health care costs have risen significantly in recent years with no sign of leveling off. There are a number of causes for this; among these are the following:

Cost of health insurance: This is the largest single factor in rising health costs, and I will discuss it in more detail below.

Administrative costs: The insurance industry is the largest source of health care payments. At present, these payments are provided from multiple sources, each of which has its own administrative structure. The combined cost is great.

Pharmaceuticals: Pharmaceuticals are the most rapidly rising segment of health care costs in the past few years, for a variety of reasons also addressed below.

New technologies: We have seen giant strides made in diagnostic and therapeutic capabilities. Medical imaging is vastly improved (e.g., MRIs are now in their third generation). There are more therapeutic options (e.g., medicated stents to treat coronary disease and various types of minimally invasive surgical procedures). Almost without exception these advances are associated with significantly higher costs; their benefits vary from minor to revolutionary.

Public demand for access to advances: The public is more aware of health care issues. Media coverage of medical advances is often overly optimistic about benefits that new advances may provide, leading patients to ask for the latest (and most expensive) options, even though these may be inappropriate to their situation, or only marginally better than standard therapy.

Care to under-insured populations: It is not widely appreciated that uninsured persons are major contributors to the rising cost of health care. When they require health care, it is provided by emergency rooms, clinics, hospitals, doctors' offices, or other facilities and charged directly to the patients. The bill is usually not paid in full, or even in part, and the unpaid costs must be absorbed by the provider. This in turn requires that charges to other patients be increased to cover the losses. One irony in this situation is that, because major carriers have negotiated reduced charges, those for the uninsured must be increased to maintain total income.

Ancillary medical personnel and services: In past years, personnel such as nurses, trained laboratory technicians, and even lower-level patient attendants have been underpaid. This is now being corrected, but it has added appreciably to the cost of care.

Updating facilities: Aging and outdated facilities absolutely need replacing, but currently functioning facilities may also require replacement or updating because of new seismic or environmental requirements.

Recouping of prior reductions: As discussed above, providers whose payments have been reduced often feel it necessary to increase their charges to maintain their income level. This should disappear when—and if—a new equilibrium of payments is reached.

The general rate of inflation: Inflation also contributes to rising health care costs, although only to a minor degree.

The Health Insurance Conundrum: For over fifty years, health insurance has played an increasing role in paying for health care in the United States. It has permitted a majority of the population to have access to acceptable health care, but it has also excluded a significant minority from equal access. Why is this so?

To understand, one must consider certain principles underlying the concept of insurance. Basically, it is based on the premise that many persons pay a small amount regularly so that a few of the covered persons can be compensated for major losses. In other words, most of those covered by an insurance plan will pay more into it over the years than they will recover. If coverage is offered voluntarily, which is the case for individual, or non-group insurance, the individual makes his own choice about whether to participate. By necessity—and in fairness to all participants—some evaluation of risk must be made before an individual is insured, with appropriate adjustments to the premium charged.

For example, those living in heavily wooded areas with limited road access are at higher risk and should pay a proportionately higher premium for fire insurance. If individuals feel that the cost of insurance outweighs their perception of risk, they will choose not to participate, or to discontinue their coverage when rate increases make coverage no longer attractive to him. Those who foresee a definite need for future insurance will enroll and renew in spite of higher premiums, leading in time to a diminishing population with an increasing number of claims. That, in turn, necessarily leads to higher premiums when the time for renewal arrives. And the process continues. Premiums increase until the company is unable to offer coverage at all. The result is an increase in the population of uninsured persons.

When group insurance is provided on an involuntary basis and individuals *must* participate, the cost of coverage is consistently less than when individuals have the option of choosing participation. Low-risk persons, who otherwise might elect not to participate, are required to do so, even though they are subsidizing the coverage of others. Most health insurance in the United States is based on group coverage through employers or other common-interest groups. The larger a group, the more predictable group insurance hazards will be with less need for frequent premium changes. In addition, the larger the group, the less administrative costs are when compared to multiple smaller subgroups of the same population insured separately. An obvious conclusion is that the larger the plans and the fewer insurance companies involved, the more affordable and stable the insurance coverage will be.

The Pharmaceutical Conundrum: Pharmaceuticals are currently the most rapidly escalating component of health care costs. Although there is some justification for this, there are also factors that do not contribute to effective development and delivery of medications. Among these are:

Research and development costs: Development expenses have always been a necessary component of drug costs, but in recent years too much effort has been devoted to the development of "me too" drugs—that is, the creation of minor molecular variants of older drugs. These then can be promoted as "new and improved." Drug companies finance such "me too" research so that the new variants will meet legal requirements, allowing them to be marketed for specific indications. The company then advertises the new drugs widely, claiming that they are superior to existing medications when, in fact, these molecular variants often provide no real advantage in patient care.

Manipulation of a drug's patent status: The law gives companies a period of time in which to exclusively market a drug that it has developed. Patent protection can also be renewed or prolonged under certain conditions. Companies sometimes abuse this right, however, in order to prolong company monopolies and high prices.

Enhanced marketing: Direct advertising of pharmaceuticals to the public is now permitted and widely used. In the past, drug companies advertised only to physicians. Physicians are able to judge the companies' claims against the realities of clinical practice. The public cannot do this, and is at the mercy of advertising that urges them to push their doctors into giving them the "latest therapy." Some pharmaceutical companies budget more for advertising than for research and development! Almost all of the best selling drugs on the market are those that are widely advertised to the general public.

Capitalism and the profit motive: Present business ethics make profit and maintenance of stock value a high priority. There is little motivation for companies to limit profit for public good.

How Can We Control Health Care Costs? We can control health costs in a variety of ways (although some may compromise the quality of health care).

New technologies: New technologies should not be adopted unless they provide demonstrable improvement in outcome. We should not adopt an expensive technology that improves results only marginally, even though patient outcomes in a few cases may suffer.

Cost of ancillary personnel: When compensation is inadequate, as judged by training and experience, it needs to be corrected. Once parity is reached, however, remuneration should not increase beyond general inflation.

Cost of updating facilities: Construction costs are hard to control beyond the scrutiny given to any public project. Construction costs of health care projects are often significantly more than other building costs because of "special requirements." "Special requirements" should be reviewed to insure that they are in fact necessary for safe and adequate function.

The Role Of Health Insurance: Health insurance is here to stay. Nevertheless, providing insurance on a voluntary basis through a multitude of providers is expensive. In our present system, over-use of health insurance can be avoided in several ways, including shifting more of the costs to insured persons, increasing premiums and co-payments, or by reducing services while still maintaining basic coverage. Plans that provide less basic coverage but higher limits for catastrophic events may also be effective. Logically—perhaps inevitably—the answer lies in compulsory and universal health insurance, offered either by a single source or by only a few major providers. Indeed, we have models of these plans in various developed countries, including the United States. Medicare is a functioning system that covers a large group of people who are enrolled involuntarily and insured regardless of their claims history. The opportunity to compare plans and choose ones with features that best suit individual preferences is lost in this system, but must be accepted for the general good.

Administrative costs: As emphasized above, having only one or a few providers would greatly decrease the cost of insurance.

Pharmaceuticals: The pharmaceutical industry's pricing policies are the primary reason for rising drug prices. Prices can be reduced only to the extent that companies are willing to address the problem in their own way. Nevertheless, the gap between the wholesale or company price and the retail or consumer price can be addressed. Drug prices could be controlled by expanding across-the-board discounts for particular groups, by large groups negotiating with suppliers, and even by government-man-dated price ceilings. The last is difficult to accomplish politically, as the recent Medicare prescription bill demonstrates, for it specifically prohibits this. Another option is to create "formula-ries"—pre-selected lists of effective drugs. Where feasible, formu-laries will include inexpensive generic medications. Individuals who use the drugs listed in the formularies have the lowest co-payment rates. Higher co-payments are required for expensive brand-name drugs that are still under patent protection. Drugs that are not listed in the formulary will require still higher co-pay-ments. Experience has shown that these plans do help to control drug costs, although care must be taken in the few cases in which patients require expensive prescriptions so that they do not stop taking the medications because of their cost.

Delivery of health care: Although institutional delivery of health care is slowly growing in the United States, most will continue to be delivered through the well-entrenched traditional fee-for-service system. The advantages of this are geographic accessi-bility, a maximum of patient choice, and personal service. The problem with fee-for-service lies in how it is financed. Tradi-tionally, it relied on a direct financial relationship between the patient and the physician. Later the system was modified so that some or all of the costs were paid by insurance coverage. The relationship slowly changed; now insurance companies pay the physician directly, and the patient supplements this as necessary.

In recent decades, additional methods of payment and deliv-ery have evolved. "Managed care" has become a by-word. The term describes plans in which patient care is monitored, either before or after the fact, with an effort to find an optimal combi-nation of effective and economical care. The most common examples include Health Maintenance Organizations (HMOs); Preferred Provider Organizations (PPOs); and Individual Practice Organizations (IPOs).

Health Maintenance Organizations: These plans may be fee-for-service, integrated, or both. Fee-for-service HMOs function in the role of traditional insurance coverage, often with the addition of centralized facilities for economies of scale.

Integrated HMOs provide the bulk of their services through centralized patient facilities including pharmacies, imaging, and ancillary services. They also are able to bargain with their suppliers for reduced charges. In addition, it was believed that HMO requirements such as practice guidelines for participating doctors, scheduled preventive care, periodic examinations, and limited enrollment might further reduce costs. There are also economies of administration including sharing of patient registration data to speed access, and sharing of patient medical data among the different sections. Patient usage and outcome data can be accumulated to help determine cost effectiveness and trends in care delivery. Historically, these measures seemed to reduce costs while maintaining quality as compared to traditional practice, but with time the savings have not been as dramatic as was first hoped. Also, in many cases HMOs have interfered with care delivery to the point that both physicians and patients have reason to believe that this not an ideal method of controlling costs.

Preferred Provider Organizations and Individual Practice Organizations: Self-insuring associations of physicians (PPOs and IPOs) have been tried. In some cases these groups provide satisfactory results, but increasingly have failed for a variety of reasons, including lack of business acumen, or lack of a large enough patient base to sustain viable insurance coverage. Capitation schemes, in which each member pays the same amount for across-the-board coverage, have almost always proved unsatisfactory, again because of a poor business foundation or too small a group, but also because they inherently present the participating doctor with an ethical dilemma: the more care he provides to each patient, the less his net income. This perception alone may be sufficient to disrupt doctor–patient relationships.

It appears that the delivery of medical care in the United states in the foreseeable future will probably lie in a combination of fee-for-service, largely paid for through insurance, coupled with a limited amount of institutional care in larger population centers, under plans resembling current HMOs.

A Solution to the Problem of Fair and Accessible Health Care? Ideally, further increases in health care costs should be proportionate to the benefits derived. Measures should include evaluating new technologies thoroughly before paying for them with community funds, scrutinizing new medical construction projects to be sure they are built as economically as possible, and urging the media to be more moderate in evaluating new advances. Prescription drugs should not be advertised directly to the general public. We should proceed in steps to achieve universal and single payer insurance coverage, even if this does not extend to all possible medical conditions or treatment options. And finally, we must force the pharmaceutical companies to function in a socially conscious and realistic manner to help solve the world's health problems. Perhaps we cannot stop the continued increase in health care costs, but if we can do only some of these things, we still should be able to slow the process. Let us hope so.

Dr. Barnett's background includes twenty years of primary care internal medicine clinical practice; Clinical Professor of Medicine, retired, at the University of California San Francisco; former Medical Director of a regional life insurance company; and Medical Consultant to the regional office of a national life insurance company.

Why Is Universal Health Care So Difficult to Achieve in America?

Jay H. Katz

I believe that every American citizen should have direct access to medical care, the standard set by the majority of industrialized nations, and a goal sought by those in less fortunate circumstances. Why is it so difficult to achieve in this country where a patchwork of individual, employer, and governmental plans still leave more than 30% of our population completely unprotected, even in relatively good economic times?

It has generally been assumed that employers contribute to insurance plans for competitive reasons, so as to have a ready supply of competent workers. This notion goes back to World War II when Kaiser Industries first set up a large-scale plan for its employees. The idea gradually was taken up by other large corporations and eventually became the norm for such entities, a result of unions and other bargaining agents for the work force. There was never a commitment, however, and there are now increasing indications that both large and small employers cannot and probably will not continue this arrangement. This undoubtedly will create a crisis in our makeshift health care system.

Other first-world nations have centralized, governmentally directed systems providing coverage for all citizens and in some cases even for foreign sojourners. My personal observations in several European countries that have such systems leads me to conclude that the level of care is not significantly different from ours, and indeed, in some cases, the sophistication of the diagnostic facilities in outlying areas is impressive when compared to similar areas in the United States. Why then is such a program so difficult to achieve here? First, I think it stems from a long-standing American distrust of governmental control, which goes back to the foundations of our nation (read DeTocqueville, for example). But in my lifetime, there has been a marked softening in this point of view. I think it is fair to say that the majority of Americans accept the necessity of central planning in large social programs, even though we may argue about the details of its administration and funding. If we can agree that the "rights of life, liberty and the pursuit of happiness" include the right to physical security in an unpredictable and sometimes hostile natural world, then it takes only our national resolve to devise a plan for equitable medical care. Another argument against a universal, centralized health care plan is that it is inherently less efficient and more costly than competitive private sector plans. It is becoming increasingly evident, however, that administrative costs in the Medicare program are much lower than in private insurance plans.

Controlling non-administrative costs is usually achieved by limiting the available services or by "cherry-picking" the population at risk—that is, eliminating the most vulnerable in our midst. In societal terms I believe this is counter-productive. The trick is to spread the risk over as large a part of the population as possible and to work backward from that starting point to determine what we as a society are willing to spend on health care. I am not against a two-tiered system in which additional benefits can be purchased through private insurance coverage for those able and willing to pay for them. However, the entry level should provide access to all and provide basic emergency and preventive services as well as hospitalization when required.

We take pride in the fact that despite the present system's shortcomings, this country is among the leaders in medical science. Many fear that a centralized health plan would produce a rigid bureaucracy unable to respond to advances in medical knowledge and treatment practices. I do not think that need be so. We should be able to devise a plan by which the unselfish recommendations of medical professionals are made an integral part of policy making. This could be done through non-governmental task forces appointed by various professional organizations. There should be room for reasonable financial reward for innovations and entrepreneurs, though it is my feeling that this was not the driving force behind medicine's achievements in the last century. In this regard, it must be asked if we as physicians can accept certain limitations to our own economic interests. There is no doubt that many of us, including myself, found the notion that we could "do well by doing good" an appealing prospect when we made our career plans. But, I believe, few of us made this the primary reason for choosing our profession. Some of us were driven by intellectual and scientific curiosity. Others by altruism. However, I think that all of us had a need to be somehow useful in the service of mankind. To aid in the goal of a rational health care system would be our second opportunity to fill that need. It can be done if only we have the wit and patience to sit down together with our fellow citizens and work it out.

Following medical school, Dr. Katz trained in internal medicine at Boston City Hospital, followed by further study in protein chemistry and a hematology fellowship. He then worked for three years as a Clinical Investigator at the Boston Veteran's Administration Hospital. Dr. Katz has served as Professor of Physiology at Tufts and later in Nuclear Medicine at Mt. Sinai in New York City. After leaving academic medicine, Dr. Katz spent twenty-three years practicing as an internist in a small town in the Berkshires. He retired in 1998.

Health Care for the Twenty-First Century

Jerome Liebman

When we began our studies at Harvard Medical School in 1949, most of us knew little about the health care system in the United States. We knew only that we wanted to be physicians, to heal the sick, to become medical investigators, to give optimal health care to all. Few of us really knew what we were getting into. World War II had ended and many of us had served in the armed forces. The country was certain that we were the best people in the world, and, having defeated the totalitarian societies we believed that we could accomplish anything. That we were a "have and have-not" society was less evident then than it had been during the great depression. That we were still a country very much divided racially was discussed but not dealt with. That access to health care was not available to all was not considered an issue. During the depression President Franklin Roosevelt initiated discussions about health care for all, but elected not to pursue it on a political basis, preferring to develop a Social Security System. After the war, we believed that everyone would have a job and that every employer would provide health insurance for every employee. If the employee was an autoworker, for example, this concept worked extremely well, and provided, at that time, a model for the country.

By the time we graduated the public consciousness had begun to change. Increasing numbers of the elderly had no job and thus no health insurance. As residents in our chosen fields, we still were not truly cognizant of the issues—our job was to get through our long residencies and get to work. After completing our residencies and fellowships, we went to work. Most of us still did not appreciate that our health care system was far from optimal.

A major breakthrough came in 1965 with President Lyndon Johnson's Medicare Bill that gave quality care to all retirees at a low cost. In addition, the Medicare Bill had built into it the funding of hospitals to provide training of physicians, salaries for house officers and improved salaries for young academic and hospital physicians.

The Medicare plan ("single payer") for all of the elderly was (and remains) remarkably successful. Medicaid for other economically challenged persons was less so. Our market-driven philosophy of health care remained, and even worsened over the next two decades, despite remarkable advances in health care in so many areas.

Writing for Americans For Democratic Action (ADA) in 1972, I provided a plan for a National Health Service that crossed state lines. When the plan was presented, the issues included optimal quality of care, inequalities of care, and maldistribution of access to good medical care. In the ADA plan the problems of today were predicted and the methods of solving such major issues as maldistribution were suggested as well as methods for cutting costs. Unfortunately the country wasn't interested in any change in our health care system. Then in the mid- to late 1980s, the media and the public finally realized that there was a health cost crisis as the technological revolution took off. The country then watched the "health care industry" grow and the media, the insurance companies and the health care industry won the battle for the hearts and minds of Congress, and of the public as well. As is now obvious, the public lost! Today our fragmented market-driven health care system is in crisis and in urgent need of radical restructuring. I still give talks about the 1972 ADA plan. I will discuss the plan below.

Although some of our citizens receive superb care, our free market has never effectively delivered optimal, humane health care to everyone at a reasonable cost. Piecemeal reform of free market health care system too often corrects one problem only to create another. A 1987 paper in the *New England Journal of Medicine* asked rhetorically whether doctors were prepared to work for corporate masters, to face ever spiraling costs, and to be deluged with complex reimbursement programs.[1] The article predicted chaos unless we adopted a rational single payer form of national health plan. The same issue of the *NEJM* also included an editorial by Editor Arnold Relman that pointed out the need for a national health plan.

By the end of 2005 we were spending more than 16% of our gross national product on health care, while Canada, which gives comprehensive care for all, was spending less than 10% of its gross national product. Yet more than forty-five million Americans, including many children, have no medical insurance, and another thirty-one million are underinsured. Many expectant mothers have no prenatal care. The chasm between the quality of life for the affluent and the poor is widening, as is the quality of health care. Care is also poorly distributed geographically, especially in rural areas. At the same time, rising costs of the mismanaged care system worry middle class and upper middle class families as well as the poor. The average private insurance company charges twenty-five to thirty cents to pay a dollar's worth of claim; they do nothing for the health care system except to limit care. In contrast, Medicare in every state charges less than three cents to pay a dollar's worth of claim. This is because Medicare is a single payer system and is thus extremely efficient. Yet Medicare is endangered by ill conceived "reform proposals" and a lack of understanding of the issues by the public. (Even if one does not wish to discuss the issue of equality of care on the basis of liberal thought, one must opt for a single payer system on the basis of economy.)

It is not only social activists who think and talk in the above vein. Gale Shearer, director of Health Policy Analysis of the Washington office of Consumers Union, wrote a paper for Consumers Union published in 1996 that provided an excellent summary of the problems faced by those with marginal incomes when illness occurs.[2] Even though families believe that they have satisfactory insurance, deductibles and co-pays are often devastating to them. With the sick paying a disproportionate share in the health care market place in the 1990s, the underinsured faced economic hardship and distress with often disastrous consequences. It is probably worse now. In 1996 for example an estimated eleven million non-elderly American families spent more than 10% of their income on health care.

The last and most inappropriate thing we need in the country is a privatization of Medicare as proposed by President Bush. We also must not be fooled by those who propose "Universal Health Care" but who recommend complicated plans including means testing which utilize private health insurers. The Clinton plan, for example, a disaster for many reasons, utilized private health care insurers, adding greatly to the cost. In an appropriate single payer health plan, there is no way to have multiple tiers, which are inherently unfair as well as expensive. Means testing as part of the system is also unfair and expensive.

Thus the only people who would benefit from privatizing Medicare would be the private health insurers, but they are so inefficient that the benefit might not be that great. The wealthiest of Americans might not be hurt too badly, but those with marginal incomes might suffer even more than now.

In 1996, before the Balanced Budget Act of 1997, there were eleven million uninsured children. The Children's Health Insurance Program (CHIP) was designed to insure half of them in five years. But with each state's economy so poor there are still close to eleven million uninsured. Meanwhile, the elderly are having more and more problems as the present Administration and Congress attempt to privatize and make it easier for the companies to insure those who are well. The new Medical Savings Accounts (MSA) are for the affluent well. (This will be discussed below.)

In 2003 we wrote a position paper, entitled "Dangers to Medicare."[3] Included in the paper were the following:

President Bush, when he first announced that he wanted to privatize Medicare, was heavily criticized from many sides. Perhaps as a mechanism for hiding the concept, in a speech to the American Medical Association in March 2003, he presented a plan, not yet completely formed, for drug benefit for seniors. It was actually a veiled plan for privatizing Medicare. Under President Bush's plan, seniors would have three options, each with different costs. First, the senior could remain in "traditional Medicare." There would be a small subsidy for prescription drugs, and the government would pay for costs above a very large amount. The second and third plans would utilize private health insurers. "Enhanced Medicare" would allow beneficiaries to enroll at varied costs in a variety of competing health plans which would include expanded coverage, comprehensive prescription drug benefits and a limit to out-of-pocket expenses. The third plan, called "Medicare Advantage," is a managed care plan in which prescription drugs are provided by the HMOs with care provided by a specific network of doctors and hospitals. For plans two and three the costs to the beneficiary would be much greater. Profits to private health insurers would presumably be built in since there would be subsidies to the private health insurers. The details for the costs of these three plans to the country and to the beneficiaries are not available as of this writing; however, there is no question that they are going to be expensive and the costs over the years would keep increasing depending upon the needs of the insurance companies. The results are likely to be disastrous. (The final plan, passed by Congress, was somewhat different, but the principles are the same.)

In traditional Medicare, seniors could go to any physician or hospital, but in order to have a meaningful prescription drug plan, as described above, the patient would have to join private health plans, numbers two or three. The small subsidy and the cap on drug costs after large amounts of money have been spent would not help for many reasons, including that many seniors would not have an initial large amount of money to spend. Further, there would be nothing to stop private health insurers from continually raising their fees in order to extend their profits. As stated by Congressman Stark, seniors would once again (as before the enactment of Medicare in 1965) be at the mercy of the "for profit" health insurance industry. It didn't work then and it won't work now. Elliot Wick of the Economic and Social Research Institute recently wrote of "risk segmentation" where patients are divided into small risk and high risk pools. Many seniors with marginal incomes fall into the high risk pools with negative consequences. The private health insurers obviously do not want the patients in the high-risk pools.

As specifically delineated by *Public Citizen* in January 2003, and as stated above, traditional Medicare is more efficient than are private plans. The Inspector General of the Department of Health and Human Services has found that, far from being as efficient as President Bush would like to have us think, private plans, even for those patients not yet old enough for Medicare and thus healthier, cost significantly more than does Medicare, with fifteen percent administrative costs instead of two percent. From 1998 to 2000 federal payments to Medicare HMOs exceeded the costs that the program would have incurred for treating patients directly in traditional Medicare by an annual average of 13.2 percent. In 1998, the program lost 5.2 billion dollars in overpayments to HMOs according to the General Accounting Office (GAO) and these overpayments continued throughout 2001. The report from Citizen Action continues:

"Medicare is more effective at controlling costs even for the elderly than are insurance companies that mainly cover the under-65 population, where price competition between plans is the norm." In fact, for services covered by both Medicare and private insurers, average annual costs of enrollee spending by Medicare has increased less quickly than for private insurers. From 1970 to 2000, private insurers posted a 10 percent increase per year as opposed to a 9.4 percent increase in the Medicare program, according to Urban Institute analysts. (For the purpose of this comparison, increases in costs for services not covered by Medicare but covered by private insurers including prescription drugs, have been removed.) If the comparison included the cost of covering prescription drugs, one of the principle drivers of increasing private insurance premiums, Medicare's comparative cost control performance would appear even better.

Ms. Shearer continues to expand upon her *Consumer Reports* paper, and in February, 2004, testified before the joint economic committee of the United States Congress. She was heavily critical of the President's concept of "consumer-driven health care," in which the problems of over-insurance were stressed rather the problems of under-insurance and lack of insurance. The president would like to see more high-deductible coverage so that the health care system wouldn't be used so much. As implied above, this kind of plan would work only for the affluent. In consumer-driven health care, costs are shifted to the sick. Yet it is well known that outcomes are poorer if adequate insurance is not available to the sick. In my own field of Pediatric Cardiology we have seen devastating results to young adults with congenital heart disease who no longer can be part of their parents' health insurance and are not eligible for the various children's programs, such as The Bureau of Children with Medical Handicaps (BCMH).

Data from the Commonwealth Fund (March 29, 1904) analyze adults aged 19 to 64 with modest incomes and in general reiterate the Fund's past documents.[4] They discussed those who had financial problems—for example, not able to pay medical bills or when contacted by a collection agency for medical bills, had to change their way of life in order to pay bills, or had major medical debt being paid off over time. Of those whose income was under $35,000, 45% of the continuously insured had problems. For those whose income was over $35,000, 29% of the continuously insured had problems. Obviously in both categories, larger numbers of uninsured and inadequately insured had even more financial problems.

A recent report (August 28, 2003) from the Health Research Group of Public Citizen points out that the United States wastes more on health care bureaucracy than it would cost to provide health care to all of the forty-four million uninsured in this country.[5] The scientific paper on which the statement was based was published in the *New England Journal Medicine*.[6] It was entitled "The Costs of Health Care Administration in the United States and Canada." The authors calculated that in 1999 the United States spent $752.00 per person more than in Canada. The Public Citizens Report upgraded the data in 2003. In the United States, administrative costs are almost $400 billion out of today's health expenditures of $1,660.00 billion dollars. Streamlining our administrative overhead to Canadian levels would save approximately $286 billion dollars, approximately $7,000 for each uninsured American. Meanwhile, other surprising data come from the Chrysler Corporation and General Motors both of whom state that a car built in Detroit costs considerably more than does the same car built in Canada. This is because in the United States very expensive health insurance has to be purchased, while in Canada that is not the case. The implications to the American economy and the automobile industry in particular are obvious.

Uwe Reinhardt, a prominent Princeton health economist, has noted that all other industrialized nations have decided that the child of a rich family and the child of a poor family should have the same chance of avoiding preventable illness or being cured from a given illness.[7] Yet as a matter of conscious national policy in the United States we still openly countenance the practice of rationing health care for millions of American children by their parents' ability to procure health insurance for the family; or if the family is uninsured, by their parents' willingness and ability to pay for health care out of their pockets; or, if the family is unable to pay, by the parents' willingness and ability to procure charity care in the role as healthcare beggars.

Meanwhile there are huge misconceptions about the Canadian health care system. The myth that great numbers of Canadians come across the border to the United States to get care is just that, a myth. There are a few wealthy people who come across, and there are occasions when a special procedure or treatment can be done only at certain hospitals in the United States, in which case the Canadian health care system pays the expenses. The latter is rare, for the major academic hospitals in Canada are of the same quality as those in the United States. Any problem that the Canadian health care system has is because of underfunding. Canada is a much less affluent country. In the year 2000 the Americans for Democratic Action (ADA) organized a conference entitled: "Health Care Justice: Building a New Movement for Universal Health Care."[8] As part of the two-day conference two speakers were physicians from Canada, Drs. Eugene Vayda, and John Marshall. Dr. Vayda, an internist and an educator was an architect of one of the first prepaid health groups in the United States, the Community Health Foundation of Cleveland, later to become Kaiser Permanente of Cleveland. Later, after a Millbank fellowship on health policy at Yale, he emigrated to Canada. He was first on the faculty of McMaster University Medical School in Hamilton, Ontario, then became a senior administrator at the Medical School at the University of Toronto where he had much to do with administering the health system in Ontario. He now runs a health program evaluation group. Dr. Vayda, who is much in favor of the Canadian health care system, states that in Canada today universal health insurance is alive and has strong popular support. Recently however the services have come under considerable financial pressure from conservative groups because of the economy, but nonetheless those groups' attempts to develop privatization have been unsuccessful.

Dr. Marshall is a surgeon, a specialist in surgical oncology. He stressed, for example, that there is a short waiting list for elective orthopedic procedures. For urgent surgery, however, the speed in obtaining the procedure is the same as in the United States. Both Dr. Vayda and Dr. Marshall gave data indicating no significant difference in outcomes related to major illness.[9, 10]

The Canadian Health Care System is run by each province with financial backup by the federal government. Key factors include:

1. Universal Insurance on equal terms for all, with portability from province to province. The care is comprehensive, including long term care.
2. The care is tax supported.
3. There are no private health insurers.

4. There is a single payer (the government).
5. There is expenditure control of volume and cost.
6. There is resource control.
7. There is technology control.

All of the cost of paying for everyone's health care needs is paid for by tax money colledted by the government. The system is nonprofit with everyone covered equally. Administrative costs are low, particularly as compared to the United States. Entry into the system and use of services is determined by medical need and not by ability to pay. The coverage is for both hospital and physician. There is no coinsurance and no deductibles. Finally it should be made clear that this system is "fee for service." The patient has his or her own physician, chosen by the patient and that physician gets paid directly by the government.

The United States and Canada are different countries with different problems. It is not appropriate for the United States, much larger, much more diverse, with much more poverty and greater disparity in the economic base of each state, to merely adopt the Canadian Health Care System. We need a single payer system designed for the United States.

The 1972 Americans For Democratic Action (ADA) plan was written for the United States and its particular problems, not for Canada and its particular problems as stated above. We are a much larger country, have much more poverty, and a much greater problem with maldistribution (i.e. disparity in the quality of health care across social and financial strata). The Physicians for a National Health Plan (PNHP) worked with Senator Wellstone (former ADA President) and developed a single payer health care system similar to that of Canada's. This was proposed for the Senate by Senator Wellstone and for the House by Congressman (Dr.) McDermott. This plan, as well as the ADA plan (and we believe any appropriate plan) must include:

1. Everyone is covered.
2. Everyone is covered equally, with equal access to care.
3. Care is comprehensive.
4. There are no out of pocket expenses.
5. Financing is from a progressive income tax
6. No private health insurance companies are involved
7. There must be a mechanism for cost containment and solutions to affect the maldistribution problem. (Actually only the

ADA plan proposes an innovative solution to help solve the maldistribution problem.)

As an aside: At the time President Clinton in 1994 set forth his health plan, ADA vigorously opposed it, as did PNHP and UHCAN (University Health Care Action Network). It was pointed out that the Clinton plan was a remarkably complicated managed competition plan, which kept the insurance companies very much in command. The insurance companies were ready to make huge profits, whereas in a single payer system, the private insurance industry is out of it. We do not have to describe what has happened since then and, given the present political climate, it is not likely that a broad universal program will be enacted soon. What the general public does not realize is that the most efficient health care system we have in the United States today is Medicare, because it is single payer. As stated above, the average health insurer charges twenty to twenty-five cents to pay a dollar's worth of claim and two insurance companies (1991 data) charged thirty-eight and forty-five cents. (It's not likely to be less in 2004 or 2005.) Yet in the State of Ohio (and in every other state) insurance contractors such as Nationwide Insurance charge just 2.5 cents to pay a dollar's worth of claim.

The ADA plan for the United States (revised very little since 1972) is most appropriate for the twenty-first century. It is expected that families (and physicians) will soon be demanding major change, and a plan such as the ADA plan would be very attractive, for it would give comprehensive care for all, at low cost, while helping us solve many problems.

We will assume a national population of 300 million people. There might be 150 academic health centers or medical center complexes, each to serve approximately two million people. Some of these academic health centers would cross state lines. Most, but not all, would include a medical school and various other health worker schools, as needed. Tertiary (complex) care would be centralized in each health center, while research and teaching would be coordinated from this center as well. Since each unit would be population-based rather than based on geography or the states, there might be six centers for New York City and environs, one for the Cleveland area, and one for Montana plus Idaho plus Wyoming together. Each medical center complex would be the center of a ring of perhaps ten secondary care units (community hospitals), which would serve a population of about 200,000 people, and where most hospital care would actually take place. But each secondary care unit would be truly part of the center even thought it might be hundreds of miles away. Attached to each secondary care unit would be multiple primary care centers where almost all care would be given (these would be the doctors' offices or primary care clinics, as indicated and necessitated by the area served). The patient would choose his or her own doctor, but that doctor, no matter how rural the area in which he or she works, would be as much a part of the medical center complex as the professor in the tertiary center. The locale and method of practice of the primary care physician would likely be different in rural areas from urban areas. The doctors in these primary care areas decide what type of office they would have whether community clinics in urban or rural areas, or typical suburban physicians' offices.

There should be no situation where optimal care cannot be given, even if the patient lives in a rural area. Any test available in the tertiary care center would also be available in the primary care area, either by computer access or other electronic means— or, if necessary, by transporting the patient. If patients need to go to the secondary or tertiary care center for tests or examination, they would get there by virtue of a transportation wing of the National Health Service. Therefore, a lumberman from Idaho or a poor farmer from Mississippi could be taken where he needs to be (perhaps by helicopter or fixed wing airplane) as readily as would a wealthy businessman from New York City. It might also be appropriate at times for health workers from the secondary or tertiary care centers to go to the primary care area.

In addition, in order to help keep all health workers up to date and stimulated, there would be frequent seminars for the health workers. Usually these would be held in the central medical center complex. Health workers would be transported to the center for these seminars.

Expensive operations, such as liver transplants or complex congenital heart surgery, would be performed at a limited number of identified "centers of excellence" thus addressing both quality of care and cost containment. Unlike what we have at present, the wealthy would not be more likely to obtain a needed organ transplant than the poor. Very specialized care units might be limited only to specific academic health units so that costly duplication, costly competition, and costly marketing efforts would be largely eliminated. If there is rationing it would be based on appropriateness of care, not on the basis of the patient's income or because the patient lives in an underserved area. There must be no "underserved areas" and everyone would have the same access to health care, whether wealthy or poor.

All of this requires control, but this control cannot be only in the hands of physicians. In fact, it would be wise to have each health unit, from the primary care center to the largest national administrative unit in Washington, be in the hands of a board of control, with each board to include health workers, health administrators, and patients. Since there is only one payment system, the paperwork mess would be much less, and it is likely that physicians would have more control of their patient's care in this system than they have today.

All health care students would get their education without cost, or with minimal cost. Determination of acceptance to medical school would be based upon the applicant's ability. The very large debts incurred by medical students today would not necessitate their going into high paying fields in order to pay back these debts. Physicians would be salaried, with an incentive plan.

In this type of Federal National Health Service the goal is one tier of care, optimal care for all. The maldistribution problem would be much less, the enormous cost of the system could be under control, and technological advances in health care could continue.

Clearly, in addition to developing a transportation wing, something must be done to control the pharmaceutical and hospital supply industries. They should not be making large profits from our patients' misfortunes. In view of the international nature of these industries, nationalization may not be appropriate, but control of the pricing structure is necessary, while allowing innovative research to continue.

We believe that the expansion of Medicare to all children offers a singular opportunity to provide quality care to a significant portion of the population and substantially reduce the long-term cost of health care. (Several national legislators in 1997 were considering preparing to address the needs of the 11 million children who are currently uninsured, but came short of recommending Medicare for Children. Instead they came up with, and enacted SCHIP [State Children's Health Insurance Program] with its fragmentation of the health care system and deepening of the current two- or three-tier system.)

Analogous to current Medicare, the system that is developed should:

1. provide a single financing mechanism free of means testing, for all children up to the age of 18, and for all pregnant women;
2. provide comprehensive care for well and sick children, including immunization, periodic screening and dental care, and other pediatric services for children and adolescents with chronic illness;
3. provide for free choice of care by individual physicians, managed care organizations or neighborhood health centers; and
4. be funded by a graduated income tax, and also by recapturing what is now being spent for Medicaid and other public programs.

The advantages of Medicare for Children include:

1. Expanding coverage beyond the poor children properly receiving legislative and media attention to include the uncovered children of the working poor as well as children from lower and middle-income families. Obviously it would cover all children. (Young families with incomes of $30,000 or $35,000 who do not insure themselves or their children because they believe they cannot afford it need to have their children taken care of as well. Medicare for Children would address this problem.)
2. Medicare for Children would eliminate the current inefficient Medicaid and SCHIP programs for children under which overburdened states often provide only episodic care, decreasing the care while the economy worsens.
3. Medicare for Children would provide an efficient payment system at minimal cost as opposed to private insurance. Thus Medicare for Children would recapture money now wasted in the health care system.
4. Medicare for Children would bring pregnant women and children to the physician early, providing well-documented improvements in health, and very likely fewer premature infants and significant cost savings.

In addition, the introduction of Medicare for Children legislation would provide a rallying point that allows people to mobilize against proposals to cut Medicare. It would curtail "for profit" control of health care. It would reduce costs for employers now providing health care benefits for dependents of workers. And, as children are a politically attractive group garnering the attention of a wide range of advocacy organizations, it is politically feasible.

The case for universal health care for children and pregnant women is both clear and compelling as well as an idea whose time has come. We join with those who champion it as the next logical step in the continuing struggle for universal, high quality, efficient and low-cost health care.

Once the country sees how successful Medicare for children is, then it will be ready to champion a single payer system of some type for everyone. The population based health plan described above would provide a rational choice.

Dr. Liebman is Professor of Pediatrics emeritus at Case Western Reserve University in Cleveland, Ohio and established the Pediatric Cardiology program at Rainbow Babies and Children's Hospital in 1960. He is politically active as part of Americans for Democratic Action as well as in other liberal organizations.

Endnotes

1. Dickman R.L., et al., "An End to Patchwork Reform of Health Care," *New England J. Medicine* 1987; 317: 1086–1089.
2. Shearer, G., "Hidden from View: The Growing Burden of Health Care Cost," *Consumer's Union,* 1996.
3. Liebman J., Fagin, D., "Dangers to Medicare." Position paper for Americans for Democratic Action, June 2003.
4. Davis, K., Health Insurance Coverage for all Americans, 1997 Annual Report. *The Commonwealth Fund,* p. 15.
5. Himmelstein D., et al., for the Health Research Group of Public Citizen (8/28/2003).
6. Woolhandler, S., et al., "Costs of Health Care Administration in the United States and Canada," *New England J. Medicine,* 2003; 349: 768–775
7. Reinhardt, U.E., "Wanted: A Clearly Articulated Social Ethic for American Health Care," *JAMA* 1997; 278: 1446–1447.

8. Liebman, J. and Shull, L., Health Care Justice. Building a New Movement for Universal Health Care—for Americans for Democratic Action, 2000.
9. Mark DV et al., "Hospital Expenditures in the United States and Canada," *New England J. Medicine,* 1993; 328:772–778.
10. Mark D.B., Naylor, C.D., Hlatky, M.A. et al., "Use of Medical Resources and Quality of Life After Acute Myocardial Infarction in Canada and the United States," *New England J. Medicine,* 1994; 331: 1130–1135.

Specialty Interests

A Pediatrician's Observations

William R. Collins

The following comments are based on the experience of a pedi-
atrician in private practice in a mid-sized city in the northern
United States.

Of all the ways in which government has influenced medical
care during my years of practice, Medicaid has been the most
beneficial. There have been many medical discoveries and technical improvements during this time, as well as a better understanding of America's health problems. It is startling today to
consider that fifty years ago sulfonamides, penicillin, and strep-
tomycin were the only antibacterial agents we had, and clinical
trials with broad spectrum -mycins were only beginning. Successful testing of the Salk poliomyelitis vaccine in field trials was
conducted in 1955. Eradication of smallpox worldwide in 1972
was a remarkable feat.

The "war on terrorism" has brought about research and study
of dangerous germ warfare agents such as anthrax and other
pathogens. Advances in radiology, with progression from fluo-
roscopy to ultrasound, and from computerized tomography to
magnetic resonance imaging, have revolutionized our diagnostic
methods. There are other amazing developments in ancillary
aids to our "old" physical diagnostic efforts. Modern medicine
has advanced at a mind-boggling pace in other ways. Many diseases have been conquered, and others have been controlled to
the point that patients can now stand to live with various chronic
illnesses and disabilities.

Advances in many other areas—ones effecting the quality of
life—are still woefully lacking. Answers to problems surrounding
payment for health care delivery remain elusive. Medicaid and
Medicare are a good start, although fiscal instability and varying
implementation from state to state have limited their effectiveness. As this essay is being written the newest attempts by the

Administration and by Congress to resolve the prescription drug problem has brought nothing but confusion—a multitude of choices with little guidance available to help individuals make intelligent choices.

The Pharmaceutical Industry: Much of the blame must be borne by the pharmaceutical industry. I admit to being prejudiced about the drug companies and their representatives—the "detail" men and women. They bombarded me during my years of practice with claims of the newest and best for their products. I never received new or original information from detail persons about any products. Theirs is an expensive method of advertising, one that fails to educate physicians. The pharmaceutical industry is rife with similar, ineffective ways in which they spend money. Recent price jumps in the cost of medications are an obvious step toward selling drugs in larger volumes under the new legislation.

Moral Considerations: Our country is in crisis. As I write these words, the horrendous tragedy of Abu Ghraib Prison in Iraq has just come to light. Blame is being passed around and one hopes that all of the perpetrators of the prison atrocities will be appropriately punished. As a World War II veteran my loyalty to my country and to our Armed Forces remains steady, but I am troubled. Do such atrocities, perpetrated by a few, indicate a moral breakdown of our society? I believe that most families are solid, intelligent, ethically sound, and morally secure. For each of those who carried out despicable acts in Abu Ghraib, I can name ten times as many hard-working, intelligent, caring, and morally sound eighteen-to-twenty-five year olds.

What part does family breakdown play in this? Is religious extremism losing sight of our society's goals? Is there a breakdown in our educational system? Has grade inflation allowed students to "excel" in a climate of dishonesty? Do television, video, and electronic games promote violence? There can be no doubt that TV (cable TV especially) and videos have had a deleterious impact on sexual mores and on respect for the feelings of others. We in pediatrics share a portion of blame for failing to educate younger generations in the dangers of promiscuity, HIV infection, sexually transmitted diseases, alcohol and drug abuse, inconsiderate behavior toward others, "runaways," street people, and unwanted pregnancies. Intensive efforts must be undertaken to address these social ills. Head Start has been a successful program, and has helped many youngsters gain a solid foundation on which to build.

Importance of Medical Organizations: I am proud of my membership in, and association with, the American Academy of Pediatrics (AAP). Unlike the American Medical Association (AMA), the AAP is dedicated to the advancement of social issues that benefit American children and also plays an important function in sponsoring continuing medical education (CME) programs. The organization is active in the political sphere, and particularly as an advocate of legislation aimed to improve the safety and welfare of children. For example, a simple observation stimulated the "Back to Sleep" program. For years physicians were taught to instruct parents of newborns to place them in a prone (tummy down) or side position to sleep. After many years it became obvious that the safest infant sleeping position is on the back. The AAP launched an intensive education program that stressed "Back to Sleep" and it has proven to be effective. This relatively simple maneuver has saved thousands of infants from sudden infant death syndrome (SIDS).

Other educational efforts have been directed at promoting good television viewing choices, wearing bicycle helmets, and the effective use of auto restraints. The Academy has notified parents and school athletic departments of the dangers inherent in youngsters' boxing or their use of three wheeled all-terrain vehicles. The AAP underwrites and publishes the "Red Book" for all practitioners. It is updated every three to four years providing the latest word on communicable diseases, immunization schedules and practices, and therapy guides for combating infectious diseases. I have found the AAP to be an excellent organization that has been a source of knowledge and teaching.

Education: Education continues to retain its position as the most important aspect of a child's development. In 1973 the 75th Congress passed the Individuals With Disabilities Act. It has undergone numerous and extensive amendments since then. Disabilities covered, types of professional help offered, and the numbers of special education teachers have expanded. During the elementary years, in addition to testing and educational evaluations, the child undergoes psychological and medical evaluations, including vision, hearing, and neurological testing. When all of the test results have been gathered, a conference is scheduled.

This includes the child's parents and teacher as well as a special education expert, a social worker, a nurse, a physician, and a psychologist, as appropriate. Test results are presented with a thorough explanation and evaluation, and questions are answered. Finally, an individualized education plan is developed, defended, and explained to the parents. The plan is then implemented, monitored, and tracked. It is also reviewed, assessed, and altered annually.

The entire process was greeted with enthusiasm in the mid 1970s and seemed to function well. Unfortunately the numbers of students increased in many areas, especially in places that have many non-English speaking pupils. There has also been an increase in cases of hyperactive attention deficit disorder, autism, depression, and similar neurological problems. Consequently, the system is overloaded and it has become difficult to provide the services required. The transition from this system to President George W. Bush's program of "No Child Left Behind" will be difficult. The Act was passed by Congress and signed by the President in January 2002. Unfortunately, funding for the program has been woefully inadequate. The overemphasis on testing will lead to serious monetary cutbacks for schools that have too many children failing the tests. The overall result will be a weakening of the finances of the most needy schools. How wonderful it would be to fund "No Child Left Behind" rather than providing unneeded tax relief for the wealthiest in our country, or to spend monstrous sums in Iraq!

Because of the demands of a global economy, children must reach high standards in order to prosper. To ensure that all children meet these high standards, we need to do much more to improve our educational system. l live in the state of Washington where students of color and ones with low income have only a 50% graduation rate. We must do better than this. Our government needs to support teachers, reduce class size, and rebuild crumbling schools. The "one size fits all" approach to testing as laid out in "No Child Left Behind" should be evaluated regularly. For example, the averaging of the tests of brilliant children together with those of students with Trisomy-21 (Down's Syndrome) skews the results in impossible ways. We need federal funds for education because the states and local communities can no longer bear the load.

Where We are Now: I have thought about changes that have occurred in pediatrics during my professional lifetime. These include the advent of fetal surgery, the separation of conjoined twins, repair of cardiac anomalies, saving premature infants with congenital diaphragmatic hernias, the treatment of necrotizing enterocolitis, and many other conditions as well. Public health specialists have done an excellent job in controlling ancient scourges: typhoid fever, tetanus, diphtheria, rabies, and epidemics of measles, polio, and other illnesses. Hemophilus influenza immunizations have practically eliminated bacterial meningitis. Pneumococcal infections, rheumatic fever, and poliomyelitis have been controlled in most civilized nations. It is unfortunate that AIDS, prion diseases ("mad cow disease," Alzheimer's, and Creutzfeldt-Jakob disease), and West Nile Virus infections have arrived to keep us alert. It is now well established that gun-related injuries are a major cause of death and injury to children and adolescents in the United States. Most of the injured are boys (approximately 80%). The majority of children who sustain unintentional firearm injuries are injured at home. The American Academy of Pediatrics urges that guns should not be kept in homes where children live, or if they are kept at home, they must be stored safely. In reality, wouldn't it be sensible to eliminate guns all together? (Unfortunately this would be difficult to accomplish, given the National Rifle Association's irrational advocacy of firearms.)

Lead Poisoning: Lead poisoning in children has been, throughout my career, a fascinating and challenging problem. The old "triple-decker" houses in the Northeast contained a veritable feast of lead-based paint, both interior and exterior. Many older communities still had lead pipes for drinking water. The addition of lead to gasoline, and lead in food and beverage containers, compounded the problem. In the 60s and early 70s, screening data found that 20–45% of the children had blood levels greater than 40 nanograms per deciliter, a level at which symptoms could appear. These children required aggressive treatment to lower their blood lead levels. Lead in the bloodstream can lead to anemia and central nervous system damage. We aimed for a level of 20 nanograms per dL. during the 1980s. Now, aggressive "de-leading" of homes, elimination of lead in gasoline, and similar measures have reduced average blood lead levels to an average of 14 nanograms per dL and 95% of children were below eight nanograms per dL. Unfortunately, the Bush Administration has put the screening level at 10 nanograms per dL. This is not consistent with good public health practices.

In Summary: I have written about recent advances in pediatrics, with special emphasis on its social aspects. I suggest that our major problems—both present and future—lie in the areas of mental health, morals, and ethics.

Following 32 years of private pediatric practice, Dr. Collins became medical consultant for the Child Protective Services of the State of Hawaii and Associate Professor in Pediatrics at John H. Burns Medical School, University of Hawaii, Honolulu, Hawaii.

Harvard Medicine in a Rural Community

Richard E. Hughes

As I sit on my deck overlooking the Tred Avon River, a major Eastern Shore tributary of the Chesapeake Bay, I reflect upon the almost 51 years since my graduation from the Harvard Medical School. The changes in the delivery of medical care in these years have been enormous—probably more than in any similar span of time since the introduction of herbal medications long ago. The changes come from many sources; some are helpful, but others are detrimental. I will enumerate some of these changes as they relate to my surgical practice in a small community hospital where I was instrumental in developing the third open-heart surgical center in Maryland, and the first such program in a non-university, rural setting.

A Community Hospital in the 1950s and 1960s: In the years after my graduation from medical school, a community hospital was a principal haven of medical care. It was virtually all things to all people, and no one was turned away. Hospital and physician reimbursement were not preliminary considerations in our approach to illness. Indigent patients were abundant and received free medical care. Doctors were frequently paid by other than dollars: a truckload of fertilizer for the garden, a bushel of Chesapeake Bay blue crabs, a catch of rockfish, varieties of farm produce, a model skipjack sailboat, a pony, a puppy from a litter of Chesapeake Bay retrievers. Malpractice suits were virtually unknown. Doctors and lawyers were friends. The administrators and other members in the vertical structure of the hospital echelon were not trained for their professional positions, but were chosen for their personalities, their benevolent qualities, and their ability to act as fund raisers for various hospital needs. There was no budgeting for research and development. Most such institutions were barely making ends meet. Physician sub-specialties were often not represented on hospital staffs. The most common specialties were internal medicine and general surgery. There were also a large group of general practitioners who had hospital privileges. The elderly population was increasing in the United States—from about 12 million in 1950 to 17.5 million in 1963. Hospital costs were also increasing, averaging about 6.7 percent each year, several times higher than the increase in cost of living. There were private health insurers on the scene, and they were compelled to raise their premiums and to reduce benefits almost annually—a difficult problem for the elderly who lived on fixed incomes, particularly in the rural areas. Two-thirds of older Americans had incomes of less than $1000 per year and only about one in eight had health insurance. Thus, community hospitals were not in a position to expand and diversify their services. Their income was also marginal.

Opportunities for Physician Continuing Education: County medical societies usually convened on a monthly or bimonthly basis. Invited speakers with a variety of backgrounds provided education. Many speakers were politically oriented and provided information to local doctors about state and national bills that involved the medical profession. Others presented medical topics of interest, public health concerns, and methods of improving health care in the community. Members of county societies were also on the local hospital medical staff. Medical staffs were fairly static with little influx of new specialties and with minimal replacements after physicians retired. Inspiration and encouragement for improvement was provided to physicians by medical specialty organizations such as, in my case, the American Association of Thoracic Surgeons, The Society of Thoracic Surgeons, The Southern Thoracic Surgical Association, and the Eastern Shore Heart Association. One could attend meetings of these organizations, converse with associates in the same specialty, listen to the presentation of countless papers on new advances for particular medical problems, and become acquainted with improved surgical techniques. It was at meetings of this type that many motivated physicians were able to assimilate changes in their specialty and become aware of advances in patient care.

Coming of Medicare: On July 30, 1965, President Lyndon Johnson signed HR 6675, which established Medicare, a social insurance program designed to provide older adults with comprehensive health care coverage available at an affordable cost. Passage of this bill resulted in drastic modifications in community hospitals. Ward services for the poor and indigent were phased out. Physicians' incomes skyrocketed although there was no increase in the services that they provide: think of the implications of this last statement. Members of our medical school class did not become physicians primarily for monetary gain. With the advent of Medicare, however, finance and business considerations intervened in the primary goal of providing humanitarian services: such was the beginning of the commercialization of medicine. Expectations of generous compensation permeated all components of medical care delivery—administrators, pharmacists, nursing staff, house staff, etc. A piece of the Medicare "pie" became available for everyone. Medical equipment manufacturers and pharmaceutical companies proliferated. Here began the long march toward what medicine is today. Included with these changes was the proliferation of various forms of treatment that eventually forced hospitals to regulate the length of inpatient stays, and brought about a rise in the number of administrative personnel necessary to handle increased paperwork. These are just a few examples of our explosive journey into the world of socialized medicine.

Changes in medical care became the byword. Medicare funds fueled the transformation of medical schools, teaching hospitals, medical specialties, and research organizations. Medicare services also served to encourage the elderly to seek more medical advice and this, in itself, brought about a mushrooming increase in medical facilities throughout the country. Without reservation, I can say that I consider HR 6675 to be the most significant change in medical practice ever introduced in this country. Yes, it does benefit many people—but, remember, that the people covered today by Medicare were formerly admitted to community hospitals free of charge and treated free of charge, and that was what medicine was all about, prior to 1965.

Next, it is interesting to note the amount of time and research expended on the development of reimbursement coding, necessary for submitting any bill to Medicare. It is commonplace for physicians to attend seminars devoted only to medical coding. Two thoracic surgical societies have combined their individual efforts and formed a "Workforce on Nomenclature and Coding." There are even coding hotlines that provide assistance to physicians who are having coding difficulties for a particular procedure. Every facet of health care service must be outlined in detail in order to receive reimbursement. This is a far cry from the days of physician compensation before HR 6675. Now, with third-party insurers the primary source of physician income, it is necessary to convince vendors of the importance and justification of medical or surgical procedures. Thus, we have introduced another element into the "science" of providing health care to our nation. As a result, the chasm between doctor and patient further widens.

Some patient groups have not been included in this system of providing health care benefits. These include the mentally ill, the uninsured, those on medical assistance, and children. These are citizens who cannot afford to underwrite the costs of political action crusades to help them gain entry to the health care system. Even so, since 1965 our nation has spent more money per capita on health care than any other western country—and we have less to show for it in terms of the general health of all of our citizens. There is no way that we can have a successful health care system until we find a way to provide for all people.

The Practice of Defensive Medicine: In the past, community hospitals provided care for all citizens, a stance perpetrated to a great degree by the generosity and dedication of the physicians on the hospital's staff—a voluntary action by physicians of the time. It was the way that medicine was practiced. Patients and physicians were on the same page, and patients were grateful recipients of the care that they received. Physicians were, indeed, "Doctors," a title far removed from the name which they would eventually inherit, i.e., that of "Health Care Providers." Thus, the doctor, a respected individual and leader in his community, was replaced by a health care "ladder" where the physician was merely one of the rungs along a complicated path.

This change in physician status was borne along by patients' expectations of consistently successful outcomes. Now, enter the legal profession! Fueled by higher patient anticipation, burgeoning financial well-being of the medical community, and the exclusion of lawyers from direct Medicare benefits, the number of medical malpractice suits increased greatly. Patient expectation has inadvertently led to an increase in dissatisfied individuals. Malpractice lawyers have reaped the benefit of discontent. The inevitable result has been an increase in the number and variety of malpractice suits. Malpractice insurance premiums have increased to the point that they cause considerable financial hardship in some specialties. Such increases have led to the early physician retirement as well as career changes.

Physicians have also been compelled to adopt a defensive approach to providing health care. No longer can the Hippocratic Oath be considered the keystone of medical practice. Anything concerning patient diagnosis and therapy now must be prefaced with thoughts of preventing lawsuits. This is strange, considering that most physicians have given their time and effort unceasingly in order to ensure successful patient outcomes. This leads to the obvious but inevitable conclusion that many malpractice claims are unwarranted, unfair, and even frivolous, bearing little relationship to an injury that was, or was not, actually sustained.

Few people could predict that such radical change would effect the life of practicing physicians. The medical system cannot sustain this level of cautious care for all. Medical insurance costs—including Medicare expenditures—necessary to support the cost of defensive medicine are astronomical. The potpourri of laboratory tests and the requests for various medical consultants that are required to protect the physician are boundless. Has any of this led to improved physician practice and better health for the patient? That, in my opinion, is doubtful. Medicine is no longer a profession. It is a business with rampant liability potential. Can medicine ever be returned to its halcyon days? That, too, is doubtful.

The Coming of Medicare Benefits to My Community Hospital: Medicare did provide the means for funding many new projects at the community hospital level. In my case, it enabled the hospital to employ a full-time cardiologist, the first "new" specialty to be introduced. The ward beds for medicine and surgery were closed. Special hospital areas were established, including an angiographic suite, coronary and intensive care units, and a special care unit. Thus, some of the ancillary services needed for a cardiac surgical program fell into place. Most certainly, without the benefits of Medicare, these improvements never would have come about.

Transition to a Cardiac Surgical Program: Many steps were involved in establishing a cardiac surgical program in our hospital—long and tortuous steps. Many individuals contributed to this project. The hospital generously provided a surgical research laboratory where we could carry out preliminary surgical team preparation. This lasted for more than two years. After final team selection and training, it was time to expose the team to a full time cardiac surgical program in an established clinical setting. This came about with the help of Dr. Denton A. Cooley of the Texas Heart Institute in Houston. With his help, our open-heart surgical team received active training in the operating rooms of the Texas Heart Institute under Dr. Cooley's supervision and guidance. Before leaving the Heart Institute on the last of many return visits, I made certain that each member of the group was thoroughly familiar with the inscription on Dr. Denton Cooley's bust in the Institute's foyer.

> "Isn't it strange that princes and kings,
> And clowns that caper in sawdust rings,
> And common people, like you and me,
> Are builders for eternity?
> Each is given a bag of tools,
> A shapeless mass, a book of rules,
> And each must fashion, ere life is flown,
> A stumbling block or a Stepping-Stone."
>
> —R. L. Sharpe

Subsequent Events: In 1972 we performed the first open-heart procedure at our local community hospital. We received telegrams of congratulations from the University of Alabama, the Texas Heart Institute, and from colleagues at the University of Maryland and the Johns Hopkins University Hospital. An adjacent bed in the Intensive Care Unit was left vacant to provide a place for team members to stay with patients during the first three postoperative days. We realized that our eventual progress in this field would depend on the successful outcomes of our first patients. Fortunately, things went well. The program has succeeded beyond my greatest expectations. A new hospital has been built. The referral base has expanded exponentially. Every possible surgical and medical subspecialty has been added to the medical staff. The reputation of the hospital has been enhanced. It is now the premium medical facility of the Delmarva Peninsula, which includes parts of Delaware, Maryland, and Virginia. Its name has been changed from "Hospital" to "Regional Medical Center" and it now serves a population of over 500,000 people. Our small, rural community hospital is now a different place. We have performed almost 8,000 open-heart procedures since 1972. The surgical team includes six board certified cardiothoracic surgeons, and we average 700 operations annually. Our team did, indeed, take to heart the message in the poem "A Bag of Tools." I can never forget the importance of this small but inspirational message; it contributed much to the success of our efforts.

Relationships with the Media: In 1972 the local newspaper had front-page headlines about the coming of open-heart surgery to the third hospital in Maryland (the first two were the University of Maryland and the Johns Hopkins University). None of the surgical team had been interviewed; the information came from other sources. Following the newspaper publicity, I received an indignant epistle from the County Medical Society berating me for seeking publicity. The letter also stated that such a newspaper article was unwarranted and unethical. I mention this to show the changes that have occurred with media coverage of medical events. Exposure in the press is now, of course, common. Physicians routinely advertise in newspapers and magazines. These undoubtedly are used by prospective patients to find "the right doctor." The internet is also a pathway for patients seeking a health care provider. In addition to physicians' names, specialties, and location of practice, one can also obtain information about credentials, education, residency training, date of licensure, as well as details about lawsuits, sanctions, dismissals, advisory letters, and other such relevant matters. Does this approach to information help physicians' reputations, or bring them more respect? I don't think so. Physicians are now just an additional rung on the health care ladder—no more and no less. Their days of leadership in providing medical care have evaporated.

The Future: I do not believe that it would have been possible to develop an open-heart surgical program in a rural community hospital after the present proliferation of medical malpractice suits. "Defensive medicine" has become the byword of medical practice. It has changed doctor–patient relationships. The ritual of informed consent is now as important as Miranda Rights that inform suspected criminals of their legal privileges. Anesthesiologists and surgeons spend more time explaining to patients their routine and their intentions than they spend on history taking and physical examinations. Laboratory procedures have become an assortment of tests to "cover the waterfront." Hospital reviewers examine patient charts to insure the adequacy of daily progress notes. Personnel are assigned to evaluate the importance of adverse medical occurrences. Physicians have even been designated as expert medical witnesses and routinely testify in malpractice cases, usually for the plaintiff. There is no end to these problems. It has helped to fragment the medical profession, limited the degree of forthrightness, and introduced an aura of suspicion among colleagues. Where will it end? There is no intelligent answer for this question. Some specialties are more at risk than others, and graduating medical students are avoiding those associated fields with known high litigation risks. The quality of these specialties may well diminish in time

Finally, would I pursue the same career path, knowing the problems that have plagued the medical profession since 1953? The answer is that medicine will always encompass both the sciences and the humanities in a way that no other profession can approach. And so I would ignore the many problems that we have encountered since 1965 and remain true to my chosen profession.

Dr. Hughes was born in East Orange, New Jersey, where he resided until entering the armed services in World War II. He was admitted to Harvard Medical School at the end of his second year at Harvard College. He served on the faculty of George Washington University and the University of Maryland. He now lives in Oxford, Maryland where he spends his time sailing and playing golf.

Science Applied to a Clinical Need

S. James Adelstein

An increasing interest in translational research has sparked a debate on how best to bring the extraordinary advances in molecular and cellular biology to the benefit of patients. How does one think about applying science to developments in medical technology? Our experience in fashioning a radiolabeled agent now commonly used in the diagnosis of coronary artery disease illustrates some of these issues.

I use the term technology to refer to devices and drugs employed in the diagnosis and treatment of disease. Such medical technologies uniformly derive from scientific advances in biology, chemistry, physics, and engineering. (The obverse is also true. The more sophisticated the experimental science, the more it depends upon technology, in the larger sense, to provide the tools of discovery.)

In general, the questions of science are designed to reveal the secrets of nature: What are genes? How do they work? What are their products? How are they turned on and off, etc.?

The questions of medical technology are designed to meet a clinical need. How can we obtain better anatomical images of an internal organ? Can we distinguish between normal and diseased tissue? Can we stage a cancer (determine whether it has spread) noninvasively?

Differences between science and technology can be minimal and, of course, many scientists are motivated to see practical benefit from their discoveries and may even participate in translating them into clinical tools. For example, studies in stem-cell biology, interesting in themselves for the understanding of development and differentiation, have obvious relevance to the treatment of failing organs such as the brain, pancreas, heart, liver, and bone marrow.

The tools of technological development are often the results of scientific discovery. Indeed, progress in the development of technologies requires a deep understanding of their underlying science. The invention of magnetic resonance imaging (MRI) required a firm knowledge of atomic properties and how to align and perturb the magnetic moment of atoms, of the interaction of microwaves with matter, the mathematics of image reconstruction, and the engineering of high-resolution magnets. Like many technological developments, it relied upon multidisciplinary activity and a good deal of technology transfer from fields other than medicine.[1]

During 1968, I took on the responsibility for nuclear medical services at the Peter Bent Brigham Hospital, and, subsequently, at The Children's Hospital, the Beth Israel Hospital, and the Dana-Farber Cancer Institute. In the job, I needed to establish not only a clinical service but educational and research programs as well. I hoped to launch a program for the development of radio-labeled agents that would be useful in both diagnosis and therapy. I immediately realized that rational progress in diagnostic agents would require knowing much more about the chemistry of the element technetium.

Why, one may ask, be concerned about technetium, that unnatural element, number 43 in the periodic table, below manganese and sandwiched between molybdenum and ruthenium? The answer lay in the peculiarities of the instruments used for imaging radioactivity in the body, in the favorable decay characteristics of technetium-99m, and in the hospital-ready supply of the radionuclide. The instrumentation developed in the late 1960s was optimized for a photon energy of 140 KeV, exactly the energy of the gamma-ray emission of technetium-99m.[2] Moreover, unlike other radionuclides favored at the time—for example, iodine-131—technetium-99m emitted no energetic particles to increase the absorbed dose to patients,[3] and its half-life of six hours confined radiation exposure to the time required for imaging. In addition, technetium-99m could be easily obtained from a hospital-based generator that could be refreshed every week instead of by daily delivery from outside reactor or cyclotron sources.

At the time, a number of technetium-99m-labeled reagents were available for patient use, but these were based on no chemistry at all or on primitive compounding methods, akin to alchemy. For the development of more specific diagnostic agents, it was clear that more had to be known about the chemistry of technetium. Moreover, as technetium is not an element naturally occurring in the cosmos, its most stable form, technetium-99 (the decay product of technetium-99m) could only be obtained in micromolar quantities.

To help with this, I went to consult with Charles Coryell at the Massachusetts Institute of Technology (MIT). Professor Coryell was an eminent radiochemist who, a victim of cancer, was happy to have his talents applied to medical problems. He recommended that a two-person team be recruited to work on the problem: Alan Davison, an assistant professor of inorganic chemistry at MIT, and Alun Jones, a postdoctoral fellow radiochemist working in Professor Coryell's laboratory. Davison would continue to work at MIT, and I would offer Jones an appointment in the Department of Radiology at Harvard Medical School (HMS). Fortunately, both seemed intrigued by the challenge of working on the chemistry of technetium and of working together as colleagues, perhaps because both had been born in Wales.

Within a year and with support first from the National Institutes of Health (NIH) and, subsequently, from the Department of Energy, the joint research was begun. The MIT Department of Chemistry brought instrumentation and graduate students to the collaborative effort, and the HMS Department of Radiology provided a source of technetium and post-doctoral fellows. Shortly thereafter, Davison and Jones produced the first crystalline product, a Tc(V)-oxo compound—one that could serve as a core to build on. Subsequently, they found that Tc(V)-oxo-N2S2 compounds were also stable, and this finding was exploited by others to produce a popular renal scanning agent.

During the 1970s, the importance of radiolabeled monovalent cations as cardiac scanning agents for coronary artery disease became evident. (In pursuit of this interest, I had spent a sabbatical semester abroad in 1976 working with an experimental cardiologist expert in the field.) The agent in common use was radiothallium ($^{201}Tl^+$), which is handled like potassium by heart cells and whose local uptake is proportional to blood flow. Thallium-201 has certain disadvantages: it is produced by a cyclotron, has to be delivered to clinics daily, and the energy of its emitted photon is not ideal for imaging.

Could one construct a technetium-containing compound that would have the same properties? Jones and Davison thought they might be able to do so. By this time they were working on isonitrile (-C=N-) complexes of technetium as Tc(I). One of these, Tc(I)TBI, a rather oily substance, was found to be taken up avidly in vivo by rat and dog hearts. When it was shown to be taken up by a human heart (mine),[4] New England Nuclear (NEN—shortly to be acquired by DuPont-Merck) showed some interest and provided a small fund to aid further chemical development. Then, sensing this research might have some commercial value, Harvard and MIT jointly filed for a patent with NEN having the right of first refusal on any useful product. In a preliminary study, 13 of 14 patients with coronary artery disease (CAD) were found to have diminished regional perfusion and decreased wall motion. However, comparison with $^{201}Tl^+$ was not favorable due to the slow clearance of Tc(I)TBI from the lungs and liver, immediately adjacent organs.

The problem of eliminating the slow lung and liver clearance was given to a graduate student, James Kraunage, to solve. Although it might be considered to be a true example of "chemical biology," it was not the kind of challenge usually given to a graduate student in chemistry. Nevertheless, the MIT Department of Chemistry allowed Kraunage to pursue it for his Ph.D. thesis. After several chemical manipulations, mostly aimed at varying the lipophilicity and other properties of the ligand, Kraunage found that esterification of the aryl groups of Tc(I)TBI produced a compound with increased clearance from the lungs and liver of animals. This agent, Tc(I)CPI, was found to produce excellent cardiac images in humans, favorable in comparison with $^{201}Tl^+$. The results were sufficiently impressive that NEN (now DuPont) paid for toxicity studies and a preliminary clinical trial in Argentina.

From this preliminary study, DuPont decided to adopt the lead compound for robust clinical use. In doing so, they substituted ethers for the esters in Tc(I)CPI producing Tc(I)MIBI (see figure), an agent that has somewhat better pharmacokinetics and can be more easily compounded in the clinic using a kit to which ^{99m}Tc is added. They gave the commercial name of Cardiolite™ to the new agent and proceeded to sponsor phase I and II clinical trials at Harvard (Brigham and Women's Hospital and Massachusetts General Hospital), Yale, and Cedars–Sinai (Los

Angeles). These multicenter clinical trials showed that Tc(I)MIBI was safe, cleared rapidly from the blood (essential in an agent that is to image the cardiac wall), and compared well with $^{201}Tl^+$ in stress-test imaging for coronary artery disease. Further studies from the same institutions demonstrated that Tc(I)MIBI could be used with single photon emission computed tomography (SPECT) equipment to obtain cross-sectional images of the heart and was reliable in detecting under-perfusion at rest (indicating that patients had previous cardiac damage) and following exercise (indicating reduced cardiac blood-flow reserve). In addition, it could be used to locate abnormalities in heart-wall motion and to measure ejection fraction (the fraction of blood in the left ventricle ejected in each cardiac contraction, a standard measure of heart muscle function).

Because of the time required to obtain FDA approval, Tc-sestamibi (Cardiolite™) was first sold successfully in Europe. Eventually it became the leading radiolabeled cardiac agent in the United States, capturing 60% of market share, despite a competitive product developed by Amersham. Over a ten-year period it generated ~$2B in overall sales, producing over $95M in royalties for Harvard and MIT, split evenly. DuPont Pharma subsequently sold its rights to Bristol–Meyers Squibb, which now spend ~$15M per year in marketing and developing new applications, such as identification of breast cancer and of multidrug resistance.

What can one extract about the interplay of science and technology in medicine from the development of this agent? Whereas, by definition, this is an example of technological development proceeding from a clinical need and resulting in a clinically useful product, it is also an example of science pursued for the same end. The scientific question asked—what is the chemistry of the element technetium—came directly from the technological requirement, unlike the classic linear model of technology development, which stipulates science first, translation afterwards.[5] It raises the dilemma of how best to bring the power of contemporary biomedical science into practical utility. Does one look at scientific discoveries and deduce which are likely to result in useful products, or does one state the clinical problem and adapt science to its solution? If the answer is both, and it surely is, then two types of skills are required; the first to see practical benefit in science pursued for its own sake, and the second to argue back from potential technology to required science.

The history of Tc-sestamibi also addresses the matter of academic university involvement in technology development. Working out the systematics of technetium chemistry is clearly an appropriate academic endeavor. How about its application to the development of a cardiac scanning agent? In some ways, the felicitous joining of a "basic scientist" (in chemistry) with an "applied scientist" (in radiology) obviates the question. Inquiry about the fundamental chemistry of technetium properly belongs in a department of chemistry as does the search for a cardiac-imaging agent in a department of radiology. But, what about a graduate student in chemistry perfecting the medical imaging properties of a compound by chemical manipulation? Should we be more careful in preserving the arena of the natural sciences in the academy? Or are we being persnickety in drawing too carefully these differences?

In tracing out the chronology in Tc(I)sestamibi development, the basic chemistry and the agent progression through Tc(I)CPI were principally supported by federal funds, whereas industry paid for the formulation of the final compound, its toxicology, and clinical trials. The patents were held by the two universities, which profited from a royalty stream. Is this what Bayh-Dole, the legislation that permits universities to hold the patents on inventions made in their laboratories under federal grants, intended? On casual inspection, it would certainly appear so. Would the work in the universities have been done without the Bayh-Dole incentive? Probably—the interest of the problem and the recognition for having solved it were almost certainly sufficient incentive for the inventors. Whether industry would have proceeded without patent protection is another matter. And, if the patents were held by industry, the universities might not have profited from the sales of product or, at least, have recovered their shares in the cost of development.[6]

In summary, this account raises a number of the issues central to bringing useful medical technologies out of university laboratories into clinical use. It begins by demonstrating the interplay between clinical need and the motivation to develop the underlying science necessary to meet it. It provides an alternative route of bench-to-bedside and shows that the identification of contemporary science in the service of medicine may not be a simple linear task.

The account also articulates the importance of integrating disciplines not only at a personal level but at an organizational

$[Tc^I(TBI)_6]^+$

$[Tc^I(CPI)_6]^+$

$[Tc^I(MIBI)_6]^+$

level as well. Institutional barriers to transdisciplinary research are well recognized,[7] and this instance of collaboration between a natural science department at MIT and a clinical department at Harvard is a tribute to breaching them. Perhaps, the practical culture of an engineering school facilitated this, although MIT is rightly proud of its accomplishments in pure science as well.

The issue is also raised as to how far in the course of development of useful products the efforts of university faculty members should be directed. In this case, the university laboratories brought the lead product to its penultimate formulation. Can faculty members be diverted from "true" academic pursuits by the promise of commercialization? And who are to judge, and how, when this has taken place? Would this useful product have been realized if a corporation had taken over its formulation earlier or would a company even have been interested?

Finally, and related to the last issue, who should profit from these discoveries and under what circumstances? This debate has raged in universities for several decades and has led to the formulation of guidelines in conflict of interest and commitment to define and contain the limits of faculty participation in commercialization.[8] At Harvard, the royalty streams are divided among the central university, the faculty involved (e.g. medical school in the case of Cardiolite™), the home department of the inventor(s), the inventor's laboratory, and the inventor(s) personally. But in this age of biotechnology, profit accrues not only from the sale of product but also from the sale of spin-offs and public offerings. How involved should universities and their faculty members be in these enterprises that capitalize on discoveries made in their laboratories, and when does participation corrupt or appear to corrupt academic values? The example given does not deal with the latter conundrum, but its resolution will be a continuing matter of debate.

Endotes

1. Once the hallmark of technology, multidisciplinary efforts have invaded the sciences of molecular and cellular biology as we try to untangle the myriad of networks that underlie the functioning of cells and of the nervous system.
2. This discussion is concerned with radionuclides that emit single photons. The development of instrumentation for annihilation photons (PET), although started at about the same time, proceeded more slowly, and the story of the emergence of this other technology is also fascinating.
3. As a result of the absorbed radiation dose delivered by the other radionuclides employed at the time, The Children's Hospital in Boston would not allow any nuclear medical procedures to be performed with its patients, other than those who had manifested cancer.
4. Dogs injected with Tc(I)TBI emit a distinctive garlicy odor. Fearful that this would discomfit patients, the inventors looked for a friendly first human subject. Much to their relief, I reported there was nothing to smell or taste.
5. In his provocative treatise, *Pasteur's Quadrant: Basic Science and Technological Innovation* (Washington: Brookings Institution Press, 1997), Donald Stokes discusses the difference between the linear model of technological development and one that sees science driven by practical need. As examples, he cites Pasteur's remarkable discoveries in microbiology motivated by the needs of the wine-making and the dairy industries.
6. One could also argue that the NIH should have received a part of the revenue stream and recovered its costs. However, this is a policy question involving the role of government in research and development, tax payer's equity, etc., and not part of the arguments I set out here (e.g. D. Korn and S. Heinig, "Recoupment Efforts Threaten Federal Research," *Issues in Science and Technology* 20(4) (2004): 26–30).

7. *Sciences and Medicine and the Physical Sciences and Engineering* (Washington: National Academy Press, 1990).
8. See D. C. Bok, *Universities in the Marketplace: The Commercialization of Higher Education* (Princeton: Princeton University Press, 2003).

Following his medical residency at the (present) Brigham and Womens' Hospital, Dr. Adelstein did post-doctoral work at Cambridge, and at Johns Hopkins Universities. He then joined the Department of Anatomy at Harvard where he established a laboratory in radiation biology; subsequently he organized programs in nuclear medicine at the Brigham, the Children's Hospital and the Dana-Farber Institute. He later served as Dean for Academic Programs at HMS (1978–98). Dr. Adelstein is presently Harvard's Paul C. Cabot Distinguished Professor of Medical Biophysics, Research interests include biophysics of radioactive decay and development of radio-labeled diagnostic and therapeutic agents.

Fifty Years without Medical Practice
Jan Wolff

Medicine: I am a bit of an outsider in these reflections because I did not practice medicine but instead devoted my time to research—first in iodine metabolism and thyroid biochemistry (this involved me in the Marshall Islands, Three Mile Island, and the Chernobyl aftermath); then I worked on protection against future reactor accidents. This in turn lead to a rejuvenated interest in potassium iodide prophylaxis against released radioiodine (thanks to 9/11). More recently I have been involved with microtubules and their biochemistry, going on to the role of anti-mitotic drugs such as colchicine, vinblastine and taxol in apoptosis (programmed cell death), and finally with cancer therapy.

I have often asked myself why I did not end up practicing medicine since many in my family did and still do; further, I was attracted to it while still young. Some reasons follow:

1. During my internship I discovered that many of the patients I saw were not, in fact, very attractive people and it was often difficult for me to develop enough empathy for them, or when I could, I felt so harassed by the load of yet-to-see very sick patients that there was no time to do anything well. That pressure was supposed to be good education, the day of the iron intern, etc., but it was not good for patients. Sometimes I could not penetrate what patients really wanted or needed. Too often there simply was not enough time to think about the problem; probably I was too slow. At other times the available remedies were dismal—the only thing for the patients with chronic severe rheumatoid arthritis in each Massachusetts General Hospital ward was aspirin—there was little interest in other drugs—patients just sat there forever, or so it seemed. I don't know how many of my fellow house officers felt this inadequacy but I certainly did. I also

resented people who woke me up in the middle of the night, more often than not about trivial problems; bad attitudes for practicing medicine.

2. It was clear to me that I did not know nearly enough practical material to do a good job. Whether or not this was all my fault or in part that of the teaching then favored at the Medical School is not clear. My daughter, who is a surgeon, did not go to an Ivy League medical school, but seems to have learned so much more than I ever did. Is this merely a function of time? Moreover, the mechanism of disease was important to me. Too often one had to act without that knowledge, one had to accept current dogma without knowing how this came about. Those who could function under these conditions were much more efficient, but I could not always accept that. Much of what we learned was, of necessity, superficial. This problem certainly has improved, and much more is understood these days regarding disease mechanisms; I would have been happy with such information. There was also a lot of confusion—I remember vividly that at the Children's Hospital it was then the fashion for the electrolyte specialists to call acids "bases" and bases "acids"—the reverse of what chemists had defined many years earlier.

3. On the other hand there is now too much information; with the present overload one wonders how medical faculties decide these days what to teach and what to leave out. I am glad I don't have to make that decision. For example, should students have to know the fascinating mechanisms by which cholera toxin, bordetella toxins (on which I once worked), or the anthrax toxins (so well worked out at HMS) cause their effects? Such aspects of molecular biology seem to be displacing the understanding of classical metabolic processes which, nevertheless, remain essential in diabetes, for example, but which are not currently fashionable. How does one deal with this? How does one avoid too much specialization resulting from this excess?

4. Some other assorted discomforts follow. With the assembly-line approach to medicine and the massive paperwork now so wide-spread in HMOs etc., my choice not to practice seems to have been the correct one even though I didn't know it at the time. I see that a number of our classmates also have sought other endeavors because of this HMO problem, or they retired early. Occasionally one can still find

a physician who will take the time to personally care for a patient's acute gall bladder or renal colic, but most won't take the time and ship the patient off to an emergency room. If a patient primarily needs to talk, forget it—there is no time for the Poloniuses of this world. While I have been lucky to be able to afford to take advantage of the tremendous advances in surgery and medicine, the price is too high for many others and their care is probably deteriorating.

5. Another medical worry is the alarming power that pharmaceutical money (grants) has in decreasing the standards of protection for patients and research subjects exposed to new, and often dangerous, drugs. This problem not only occurs at the level of the FDA, which seems to me to be severely weakened by conflicts of interest, but also in many research-type medical schools—publishing a paper seems to outweigh caution all too often, particularly if it promotes drugs and hence more grants. Publication of negative reports is often blocked. How much of this clinical research is biased by the commercial interest of the investigators? How reliable is the information? The New England Journal of Medicine seems to be making a valiant effort in this direction, but even it doesn't always catch problems. In addition, sticking a mere methyl group on some compound whose patent runs out should not constitute grounds for de facto patent extension and continuance of high prices.

Does that mean that my education at the Medical School was a waste of time? Definitely not. There simply is no way to understand the benefits and limits of medical thinking without going through it, since it is so different from the physical sciences. You can't just wait until a clear-cut answer is available—you have to act in the now with whatever poor information you have, much of which is epidemiological in nature, often with excruciatingly high p values, despite large samples. On the other hand, it has been a pleasure that in some of my work I was able to transfer easily what I had learned to a clinical environment with which I am occasionally involved. This could not have happened without HMS.

Research: In the lab it has been a great satisfaction to work and discuss work with so many smart (a lot smarter than I) scientists: they often have a completely different approach and storehouse of information and point out things I have forgotten. They clarify ideas, stimulate and criticize at the same time, and sometimes offer one the opportunity to do the same for them. In addition, I have had the privilege of working in foreign laboratories where quite different points of view come to light. These include ones in Paris, London, Lyon and Naples. While there are many failures in research no matter what laboratory you are in, there is no high like having an important insight that nobody has ever thought of before. These often involve understanding a mechanism or process or just a clue as to what to do next, allowing one to finish a study and publish, etc. While it is not possible to escape the "publish or perish" pressures entirely, the NIH has been relatively tolerant about this, permitting one to try long shots. For me the most important part of publishing is to learn what is missing in my logic and to organize my findings into a coherent whole that can't be "improved" any more. It has been a puzzle that so many Fellows find this writing portion the most difficult aspect of research, and I have spent a considerable amount of effort trying to help with this. And yet, research at the NIH has changed. It used to be enough to find out something interesting. Now such findings are relegated to the background unless some application is immediately visible; and if not, you are expected to invent some sort of relevance that will make the work appear to be useful in medicine. Since most biological processes can be related to cancer this is not too difficult, even if slightly dishonest. If a discovery is too far removed from that goal, it will not be understood. Some of the discoveries I was most pleased with weren't hot sellers, while some lesser items were very popular. So it goes. The push toward directed research seems to be unstoppable, presumably because Congress wants clinically applicable results. I know how hard it has been at times for a director at the NIH to explain research to Congress.

Finally, in many fields and in my current area of work (tubulin and microtubules) there is so much new material in the literature every day that information management becomes a nightmare and one has to become highly selective and, thus, too specialized. It gets more and more difficult to keep up. Nevertheless, I am somewhat reluctant to kiss all this good bye because I enjoy the stimulation of the research ambience so much, and I also like a certain degree of scheduling imposed on my day—not too much of that, of course. If I retire I can always complete several half-finished reviews and attend seminars, etc., but it will not be the same. Will piano and oboe playing, travel, perfecting my French and/or my Italian be enough?

Politics: The current national outlook seems depressingly bleak—the complete disregard of the future for the sake of re-election or other current purposes is utterly shameful. Have we not had enough of the flood of tiresome, banal and inane homilies, reassurances and fabrications to justify poorly thought-out political and military adventure? There is near total disregard for fiscal discipline, which unloads enormous debt on future generations; there is unchecked destruction of the environment for short-term gain—priorities may have shifted from land to oil and I assume that water may soon become more important than oil; and there continues to be appointments of politically correct but incompetent people. It is very dangerous for us and the world. The "free lunch" promise as a basis for policy has become the opiate of the American people. Nobody seems to remember the Laws of Thermodynamics: First—"there ain't no such thing as a free lunch" and second—"you get less than what you paid for."

The Administration is gravely compromised by numerous conflicts of interest (Halliburton: one wonders if anybody in Congress was awake when these assignments slipped by)—that is, self-interest—at the expense of national interest. It has needlessly offended most of Europe; provides glib and simpleminded talk of overnight democracy for everyone else (disregarding deeply entrenched tribal systems and religious division as well as the learning curve) while eroding it at home; and it appears to be bent on destroying the environment as a dowry for its supporters. This last is particularly worrisome because of a lack of reversibility as so convincingly pointed out in Jared Diamond's recent book *Collapse*. Whatever evidence unfavorable to the Administration is doctored, or pushed aside by asking for more study, that is, no action. In addition, the lack of recognition that world population pressure will impact on the United States has led to foolish restriction on birth control measures. Letting the third world die of AIDS or kill itself in wars hardly seems an optimal solution to the population problem. Population control is part of that picture and should be handled at the same time—this requires better education; the birth rate in

Kerala is a good example of how well this can work in India. One probably has to leave it to women in order to remove the male ego from the equation.

How could all of these problems have happened in the World's Greatest Democracy? Does it have anything to do with the use of power—power corrupts and absolute power corrupts absolutely? Due to my background I am sensitive to this. In order to secure power, starting a war is a successful procedure. Bismarck, the Kaiser, and Hitler are prime examples, and the lesson has not been lost on Bush—there is an almost guaranteed rush of patriotism at the beginning of such adventures. Seizing land or starting a pre-emptive war against imagined or manufactured dangers (Sudetenland, Poland) rings a bell, and the Kaiser's unshakable drive to World War I is a clear example of such abuse of power (beautifully documented by Fritz Fischer—*Griff nach der Weltmacht*—which is based on documents about the Kaiser period captured only after World War II; it has been translated into English). This abuse leads to progressively restrictive laws that are passed under the guise of emergency (the Patriot Act in our case), such that previously illegal actions are now legal; only later does legality become irrelevant. Appointment of judges becomes more and more a question of political adaptation to current dogma. Internal disagreement with the policies of management becomes treason or at least grounds for dismissal. Finally, there is the incarceration of undesirables without a trial or legal access; the last time this country had concentration camps was with the Nisei and it took a long time to redress that embarrassing injustice; in fact, a full restoration is quite impossible. Happily enough the American system's built-in inefficiency puts numerous road blocks in place against such excesses, and more and more people in the right places are finally beginning to wake up about the dangers of such adventures. The paranoia currently gripping the country, that has made this possible, will, hopefully, subside. It has subsided before, ever since the reversal of Alien and Sedition Acts. It is an interesting question how an open society should respond to a real or perceived emergency, but destroying that openness seems a high price and I am not sure we ever get all of it back. Destroyed reputations are hard to restore, exonerated prisoners are not compensated in most States (responsible justice departments and slovenly, or worse, prosecutors should be made to pay), trials should be prompt and open, jury selections should not be racist or biased in other ways, etc. The Law is far less "majestic" than it pretends to be.

So what does one do? We support the American Civil Liberties Union, Save the Redwood League, Environmental Defense Fund, Chesapeake Bay Foundation, Sierra Club, Concerned Scientists, etc. But all this is pretty passive and we feel guilty. Maybe that is why one should retire? And maybe we will!

———————

Dr. Wolff's home is in Bethesda, Maryland. He and his wife still work in the lab. He says: "It will be hard to leave, but I have not taken on any Fellows in the last year. As time allows I play the piano and the oboe. I also enjoy sailing in the Chesapeake, and downhill skiing in Utah."

Medicine and the Law

Medical Legal Comments

Max Martin Halley

My primary interest and activities have always been in medicine, with focus on excellence in the delivery of care to surgical patients. During my early years of surgical practice, I pursued the study of law as a part-time student, leading to the JD degree in 1966. Thereafter, while continuing the practice of thoracic and cardiovascular surgery, I participated in a small informal group of professionals with similar interests, aiming to improve understanding between the medical and legal professions, and later to attempt development of possible solutions for interdisciplinary problems.

The formal Midwest Institute for Health Care and Law was incorporated in 1987 in Kansas by some members of the original group. As executive director, I supervised the coordination and participated in ongoing programs—local, state, regional and national—for presentations, symposia, and publications. At this time our efforts were largely directed to the analysis and possible solutions for the medical malpractice problem, which we believed to be a major threat to medical care of patients as well as a primary source of controversy with the legal profession.

Our analyses, conclusions, and recommendations for three topics are presented in this publication. The subjects indicate the progression of our attention from general and ethical issues to in-depth focus on solutions for the medical malpractice problem. They continue to be relevant, and are presented in discussions concerning the beginning of life as well as the related issue of abortion; the moment of death; and medical malpractice, topics that reflect my "extracurricular" activities for approximately forty years.

Problems of Life and Death

Medical, legal, and public concepts concerning the beginning of human life (personhood), as well as the moment of death, have been major concerns in recent years. In past decades these concerns were highlighted by end-of-life issues in the form of potential homicide charges against physicians for pronouncing death in the presence of a beating heart. Today, concerns are focused on the beginning of life in the emotional and frequently violent confrontations on abortion.

The Beginning of Life: The time that life commences has been the subject of speculation since ancient times, when the fetus was not considered alive until some time after conception. For example, Hippocrates placed the time of fetal life at thirty days after conception for males, and forty-two days for females. Aristotle placed it at about forty and ninety days respectively. Galen placed it at about forty days for both sexes, a time also then accepted by the Roman civil law, while various other writers subsequently advanced their own speculations. Augustine in one of his writings expressed the opinion that there was a time in embryonic development when life came in, but no human power could determine this point. He later confessed that he was unable to make a final decision on this issue.

In the last of the twentieth century, the matter remained unresolved, as medical and legal concepts continued to manifest vagueness, non-uniformity. and dissimilarities. Medical authorities generally recognized life as beginning at conception, but believed that the human personality (personhood) began at viability—the time the fetus attained the capacity for independent existence—a time not precisely ascertainable. Legal authorities, on the other hand, considered both the beginning of life and the moment of death as subordinate facts, which permitted the determination of other important legal relationships. Consequently, for legal purposes, human life was considered to arise at various times, ranging from the moment of conception for property or inheritance rights—if subsequent live birth occurred—through viability or "quickening" in some personal injury actions, to the moment of live birth in criminal law, or as determined by an existing statute. Thus, the law adopted a multiphasic approach to the beginning of the legal personality, the point in time when the developing fetus was entitled to protection under the law, depending on the legal issues to be resolved. The beginning of life was therefore governed not only by the case law and statutes of a particular jurisdiction, but also by the different approaches of the law of property, the law of torts, or the criminal law.

The Moment of Death: Similar ambiguities also concerned the moment of death, since individual tissues and organs "die" at different times following cessation of respiration and circulation, and manifest different intervals during which resuscitation can be successful. Legal concepts accepted the traditional definition of human death, consisting of irreversible cessation of "vital functions," that included brain function, respiration, circulation, and impossibility of resuscitation. Medical views, on the other hand, while ordinarily based on similar criteria with clinical emphasis on the absence of a heartbeat, were additionally adopting cerebral criteria—the irreversible cessation of brain function—for the pronouncement of death even in the presence of a beating heart. This conflict between the established legal definition and the new "extraordinary" medical concept of brain death involved potential allegations of homicide. The legal moment of death was therefore an important medical consideration in life support decisions, resuscitation procedures, or in the harvest of organs for transplantation.

We addressed this issue in several articles, beginning with " Medical vs. Legal Definitions of Death" (Halley and William F. Harvey, *JAMA* 204, 1968), proposing a uniform definition which would include brain death, and which would be acceptable in both medicine and law. Kansas subsequently, at least partially as the result of our efforts, became the first state to adopt a statute defining cerebral death, a concept that presently has become generally established.

Life and Abortion: The abortion issue, centered on the definition of when "life" begins, presently a major area of disagreement, involves religious convictions, church edicts, concepts of morality, and political maneuvering. It must be viewed in the context of current improved survival in prematurity and presently available imaging or monitoring techniques, which permit better identification of intrauterine development.

In the 1960s, American law, reflecting English law, still regarded interference with pregnancy as criminal, unless performed for therapeutic reasons. These reasons, however, frequently lacked clarity and most commonly referred only to the life of the mother. In that era, compulsory sterilization for the feeble minded was still the law in twenty-seven states, eighteen states had compulsory sterilization laws for the "insane," and a child produced by artificial insemination with semen from a third-party donor might be declared illegitimate or even result in allegations of adultery. Contraception, too, was frequently prohibited by law, and the sale of contraceptive devices in some states was permitted only for prevention of disease. Pressures for reform were widely evident and many changes resulted from the repeal of statutes or court decisions. Presently, however, the pendulum appears to be swinging toward increased restriction manifested by federal government opposition to contraception, abortion, and stem cell research, as well as by legislation and religious pronouncements.

In Kansas, my colleagues and I recommended liberalization of the abortion statutes. We discussed several alternatives, including the Kansas Medical Society recommendations. These proposed to remove abortion from the criminal law, with subsequent supervision through the administrative and professional controls existing in licensed and accredited hospitals. Then, the United States Supreme Court dramatically changed the abortion landscape in the historic decision Roe v. Wade (1973). This decision established a standard of permissible controls of abortion, ranging from prohibition of state intervention to increasingly permissible controls as the pregnancy progresses: in the first trimester the abortion decision is left to the pregnant woman and the medical judgment of the attending physician; in the second trimester the state is permitted to regulate abortion in ways reasonably related to maternal health; subsequent to viability, the state may regulate or even prohibit abortion except where it is necessary in appropriate medical judgment for the preservation of the life or health of the mother.

The battles over abortion are still in progress and are intensifying. The problem is fundamentally one of definition, concerning the point in fetal development when society and the law will recognize "personhood" in the fetus. It is, however, also a problem concerned with a woman's right to control her body, encompassing the risks to her life or health, or the equally difficult considerations of severe fetal abnormalities, rape, or incest. In the past, older men have made reproductive rules for young women in the name of morality or religious doctrine. Although this patriarchal culture still persists, there is now substantial support for a woman's right to choose, most likely within the Roe v. Wade framework. In my view, this is primarily a women's issue: women, having won the suffrage battles, must now exercise their voting rights at the ballot box and thereby determine whether their right to choose should continue, be restricted, or be abolished.

My own support is for "choice" as outlined in the Supreme Court decision, grounded in the belief in equal rights for women, personal experiences with the results of "coat hanger" abortions, and in the conviction that government should not be unduly intrusive into medical decisions between patients and physicians. However, it is incumbent on women, who represent a powerful voting block, to determine this issue. Should women be indifferent, they will nevertheless be bound by the results. Moreover, any legislation, whether state or federal, will be unsatisfactory since a dominant group will thereby impose its subjective views on a substantial minority with different beliefs. The criminal law particularly seems inappropriate for these problems, since resolution by other means is entirely possible: the issues can be addressed as any other medical condition within the patient–physician relationship, subject to the established quality controls in accredited health care institutions and the supervision of licensing authorities.

Conclusions: The beginning of life and the moment of death are definitional problems. They are arbitrary points in human development and human exodus, requiring clarification based on medical evidence, societal acceptance, and ultimately approval by the law. The moment of death, which generated considerable controversy in the 1960s, is not presently problematic. The moment is a medical determination and is ordinarily established in an unresponsive individual by irreversible cessation of the circulation evidenced by lack of heartbeat. Death may also be pronounced when total brain function is irreversibly absent even in the presence of continued function of other organs.

On the other hand, differences continue concerning the moment when life begins—the point in human development when the fetus is recognized as a legal person. While a universally applicable and uniform definition may not be possible for this event, a point in gestation established by societal consensus seems possible. This approach should minimize or ideally avoid intrusion of the criminal law into the course of pregnancy, allowing highly personal and critical decisions as in any other medical condition.

Medical Malpractice: Solutions for Injury Compensation

The frequency and severity of medical malpractice claims have increased dramatically in recent years, and have continued to affect the medical practice environment adversely. This has not only been a major disturbance in health care, but has also resulted in crises in the 1970s and 1980s, and another developing crisis at present. Each crisis was triggered by increasing cost and decreasing availability of physicians' liability insurance, with greater severity in some areas of the country and for some medical specialties. Since physician costs have been the main driver in the development of these crises, remedial action by legislatures and Congress responded with tort reforms generally designed to make the bringing of a lawsuit more difficult and decreasing the amount of the award if the suit is successful. This pattern of response may be compared to moving trees into different positions in a forest, while ignoring the expanse and continued growth of the forest itself. Thus, although each crisis subsided following the implementation of tort reforms, these have yielded only temporary solutions prior to another exacerbation of the continuing problem. Moreover, the tort reform solution has ignored other important aspects of this many-faceted problem, such as the detrimental impact of the adversarial litigation process on the general medical practice environment, destruction of the physician–patient relationship, and effects on physician practice patterns. It has established quality assurance focused on a minor cause of malpractice, the "bad doctors," thereby diverting attention from the fundamental serious problems negatively affecting the delivery of health care. And most importantly, it has not addressed the role of inefficient compensation of injured patients through the legal lottery. This lottery, under the present tort system, requires patients with real or perceived injuries to proceed against providers in a slow, uncertain, expensive, and adversarial process in which there is an occasional big winner while many others receive no compensation. The entire process of claim resolution may take several years, and is emotionally traumatic for providers as well as patients.

After several years of discussion and extensive research, we believed that an alternative to the tort system, an administrative process rather than adversarial litigation, would present the greatest probability of a permanent solution. We evaluated the proposals of legal scholars as well as several existing compensation systems abroad, and again concluded that the traditional tort system was unsatisfactory even with standard tort reform. Moreover, an administrative no-fault compensation system for all adverse events was also unsatisfactory, since this alternative appeared prohibitively expensive and unnecessary. The proposed "intermediate" solutions all retained parts of the tort system, but appeared to present significant advantages to the extent that they departed from tort law and the court-based litigation process. Several administrative systems, moreover, were functioning in other countries, and in Great Britain a different application of the tort system was yielding less controversial results. A comprehensive administrative system for application to this country, however, did not exist, although others had previously discussed the concept.

Our project, therefore, became the development of a model medical accident compensation system analogous to workers compensation programs, whose track records in every state could serve as guidelines. With the initial support of the State Medical Society, a former director of the state Kansas Workers' Compensation Board was retained in 1985 to draft a prototype statute, which was later modified by us and published. Our proposed administrative system eliminates the adversarial confrontations inherent in tort law and litigation, defines health care injury, provides prompt and fair compensation based on health care error without requiring the determination of individual fault, and includes comprehensive quality controls. The completed statute received favorable comment from several reviewers, and was introduced into the Kansas legislature in 1989, where it did not progress beyond the Insurance Committee.

A number of presentations and several publications resulted from this project, including our book, *Medical Malpractice Solutions: Systems and Proposals for Injury Compensation,* Halley, Robert J. Fowks, Calvin C. Bigler, and David D. Ryan, eds., Charles C. Thomas, 1989). Chapters of the book discuss each proposal for solving the medical malpractice problem, whenever possible by the original authors in this country and abroad, with additional contributions by other scholars and the editors. Contributions also discuss the history and development of tort law and its impact on health care, the status of professional liability in the United States and in Britain, the economic evaluation of the compensation system, and the constitutionality of medical malpractice reform legislation. A final article, "Towards a Solution to the Malpractice Problem" (*Surgical Oncology Clinics of North America* 3, 1994), summarizes the material, and represents our final effort prior to dissolution of the Midwest Institute for Health Care and Law.

Conclusions: The available options for solution of the medical malpractice problem can be considered as a spectrum, ranging from unreformed traditional tort applied to all claims, to administrative no-fault compensation for all adverse events. Intermediate solutions, each revising the tort approach to some degree, present significant advantages to the extent of their departure from tort law, adversarial litigation, and jury verdicts. Tort reform, the standard intermediate, which has not provided a lasting solution and has not prevented recurrent crises, nevertheless remains the only option seriously considered by the medical profession and other concerned entities. Until sufficient support develops for trial of another alternative, the hostile atmosphere of tort litigation will continue to plague the profession while hindering the compensation of injured patients. "Fault . . . liability . . . adversary . . . litigation . . . ," the essential foundations of tort substantive law, presently still persist. We must hope that these foundation concepts of tort law will in the future be replaced by an administrative system, based on consumer-oriented compensation for injury rather than emphasis on provider economic relief. Such administrative compensation, however, cannot be a panacea, since determinations may still be subject to disagreement, insurance premiums will still be necessary, and quality review proceedings will still occur. Nevertheless, the Model Accident Compensation System appears worthy of a field trial in one or more states, since it incorporates the best features of the various proposals, and appears most closely to approximate the essential criteria for long-term resolution of the medical malpractice problem.

Dr. Halley was born in Germany, the son of family physicians. Following surgical training, he practiced general, cardiovascular, and thoracic surgery in Topeka, Kansas, from 1959 to retirement in 2001. He received the JD degree from Washburn University School of Law in 1966, subsequently serving as Lecturer in Law at Washburn; Assistant Clinical Professor of Surgery and Associate Clinical Professor of the History and Philosophy of Medicine at the University of Kansas. Dr. Halley was a founder and director of the Midwest Institute for Health Care and Law. Since retirement he has pursued interests in history, religion, and general education studies.

Physician Aid-in-Dying

Ralph D. Tanz

Phil was diagnosed with mesothelioma, an aggressive and painful disease generally caused by extensive exposure to asbestos. Recommended treatments were of no avail. He confided to his wife Joan that he wanted to end his life and asked her to help. Under tremendous emotional pressure, Joan called upon Oregon's office of Compassion in Dying. Several advocates from the office came to their home and explained the process to Joan and Phil, reassuring them that Phil was qualified to use the law since his two physicians agreed to cooperate.

On the day Phil decided he was ready to die he asked Joan, two close friends, and two Compassion volunteers to be with him. He asked his friends and volunteers if they would please step into the other room while he and Joan spent some time together. He then climbed into bed. After a short time Joan called everyone back into the room. Phil drank the mixture quickly and asked his wife to curl up next to him. He took her hand and said, "I love you." Within a few minutes Phil died as he wished—with dignity and grace.

History and Details of Oregon's Death with Dignity Act

Since November 1997, Physician Aid-in-Dying has been legal in Oregon. The Oregon Death with Dignity Act, a citizens' initiative, was first passed by the voters in November 1994 by a 51% to 49% margin. Immediate implementation of the law was delayed by a legal injunction. After many legal proceedings, including a petition to the U.S. Supreme Court, the Ninth Circuit Court of Appeals lifted the injunction in October 1997. Oregon Measure 51, placed on the November 1997 election ballot, asked voters to repeal the Act, but was defeated by a 60% to 40% vote. The Act has been tested in the courts and upheld by the federal court. Efforts by several members of Congress have also tried to suppress it, but the promise of a senate filibuster has defeated those efforts. More recently former Attorney General Ashcroft attempted to punish doctors who prescribed drugs using Oregon's law, but a federal court issued a permanent injunction against him. Nevertheless he has appealed that federal court ruling to the Supreme Court and the outcome is uncertain. The Death with Dignity Act allows terminally ill Oregon residents to obtain from their physicians prescriptions for the self-administration of lethal medications. Further, the Act also states that the ending of one's life in accordance with the law does not constitute suicide. Although the Death with Dignity Act legalizes physician aid-in-dying, it specifically prohibits euthanasia. The purpose of the Act is to restore control of end-of-life care to the patient. To comply with the law physicians must report to the Department of Human services all prescriptions for lethal medications. In 1999 the Oregon legislature added a requirement that pharmacies must be informed of the prescribed medication's ultimate use. Oregon law, as well as the American Medical Association's guidelines, also state that a health care provider shall not be required to write a prescription to end human life (Oregon Death with Dignity Act, Section 4.04).

Who is Eligible? The law requires that the patient: be an adult (eighteen years of age or older); be capable (mentally competent); able to make and communicate health care decisions; be an Oregon resident; have a terminal illness (defined as a disease that will, based on reasonable medical judgment, produce death in 6 months); and, finally, make a voluntary request.

Ethel was one hundred and three years old. She lived in a nursing home with her husband, a victim of Alzheimer's disease who no longer recognized her. Although her eyesight, hearing and writing were quite good, she needed the nursing staff full time because she was confined to bed and required assistance with her bodily functions. Her weight had shrunk to seventy five pounds and her legs could no longer support her. Ethel decided that her quality of life was no longer acceptable and she no longer felt like living. She therefore inquired as to whether Oregon's physician aid-in-dying law might assist in helping terminate her life. But since Ethel did not have a terminal illness she was told that she was not eligible. Whereupon she announced that she would cease eating and drinking. Four days later she slipped into a deep sleep and died shortly thereafter.

Legal Requirements of the Attending Physician: If the attending (or consulting) physician believes the patient may be suffering from a psychiatric or psychological disorder or depression causing impaired judgment, an evaluation by a psychiatrist or psychologist may be required. Should the patient be deemed not to have a mental disorder influencing judgment, a physician can then write a prescription to hasten death. At that time the physician must document the elements of an informed decision as follows: diagnosis, prognosis, potential risks associated with taking the medication, result of taking the medication, and the feasible alternatives, which include but are not limited to comfort care, hospice, and pain control. In order to protect all parties, documentation must be provided that the patient has been reminded of the right to rescind the request, discussed his or her intention with close relatives, and that the patient take the medication with another person in attendance in a non-public site. A consulting physician must confirm the diagnosis and prognosis.

The consultant must examine the patient and relevant records and explore the issues that form the basis of the patient's request. Documentation is required to confirm that the patient has a terminal illness, that he or she is capable, is acting voluntarily, and has made an informed decision. The consultant may request a referral to a psychiatrist or psychologist as well.

Timing Safeguards of the Act: The attending physician must wait at least fifteen days after the patient's first oral request and forty-eight hours after the patient has signed the Request for Medication form to write the prescription. The patient cannot sign the Request for Medication form until the attending and consulting physicians have determined that the patient is terminal. The patient may make the second oral request no less than fifteen days after the first request. Both the attending and consulting physician are required to submit forms to Oregon's Department of Human Services. The Department's sixth Annual Report noted that 208 patients between 1997 and 2004 have successfully hastened death by ingesting a barbiturate according to Oregon's law compared to 53,544 Oregonians dying of the same underlying disease (see attached table). Of the 208 patients, 87% (180) had either cancer or amyotrophic lateral sclerosis (ALS). Although the number of Oregonians ingesting legally prescribed lethal medications has increased, the number of terminally ill patients ingesting a lethal medication has remained very small (0.39%).

Opponents of the law frequently argue that pain is the real reason why patients seek a hastened death. But studies confirm that it is the loss of autonomy and not pain that motivates terminally ill patients to explore assisted dying as an option. The three most often mentioned reasons given to physicians are the loss of autonomy, decreasing ability to participate in enjoyable activities, and losing control of bodily functions. These findings are supported by a recent study of hospice nurses and social workers caring for PAD (physician-assisted death) patients in Oregon. Hospice care has been touted as an alternative to PAD. It turns out that, of the 208 persons in Oregon who died by physician-assisted death between 1998 and 2004, 178 (86%) were enrolled in hospice programs. Enrollment in a hospice program does not appear to be a barrier to requesting and receiving a prescription for a lethal medication. Oregon patients possessing a college degree and those with higher socioeconomic status are more likely to chose PAD. Possibly those individuals are more knowledgeable about end-of-life choices. Patients requesting assisted death were described by physicians as being determined and inflexible. They wanted to avoid dependence on others and were described as being outspoken, articulate, single-minded, mentally competent and intelligent.

It is also important to realize that patients with a disease such as ALS in which the inability to work, engage in pleasurable activities, care for oneself, and communicate, constitutes such a formidable loss of autonomy that they want to control the means of their death. "I don't want to linger and dwindle and rot in front of myself—I want to go out with some dignity. And I want my friends to be there." The Death with Dignity law included a proviso that patients requesting a lethal medication might have to prove mental competency to psychiatrists or psychologists. This has given rise to a number of questions. Was this requirement placed in the law so that psychiatrists and/or psychologists should act as gatekeepers? Was it done so that Society would be "let off the hook"? Was it done to insure that major depression was not playing a role in the patient's request for PAD? Does the wish to commit suicide infer mental incompetence? Was it included to "disguise society's ambivalence about suicide itself"? Some courts have stated that the presence of a mental disorder does not automatically infer incompetence to make medical decisions. In 1996 Ganzini and colleagues reported that Oregon psychiatrists varied considerably in their confidence to determine competence in one or more consultations. But what are the standards for determining whether a patient requesting PAD is competent? It has been suggested that the ethical views of psychiatrists could influence their opinions regarding competence. Proof of competence should be "clear and convincing" and "beyond a reasonable doubt." A very stringent standard should be used to determine competence. Some psychiatrists argue that depression causes impaired judgment and that mental disorders are strongly associated with suicide. And it is claimed that the desire to die for most suicidal patients is not permanent. But are these arguments sufficient if the depressed patient has less then six months to live? The point at which the disease process affects a person's mental ability to give informed consent is nebulous. Depression obviously is common among patients considering PAD. (It was of interest to learn that about 20% of patients who are either terminally ill and not suicidal, or just depressed, consider PAD.)

Discussion: Some members of our society believe that, depending on the situation, an individual's personal freedom should be abridged or even cancelled; that human life is sacred and that it is immoral or unethical to terminate it themselves. Yet these same people would not hesitate to "put down" their suffering pet. Many who are religious feel that mental or physical suffering is secondary to maintaining life regardless of an individual's wishes. An unwillingness to participate in PAD has been associated with religious beliefs, especially Catholicism. Responding physicians with no religious affiliation were most supportive of PAD, while Catholic physicians were least supportive. Religious preference was the only variable significantly associated with either favoring or opposing legalization of PAD. Nevertheless, other physicians may question whether PAD poses a threat to the profession of medicine and their obligation to "do no harm." It is when religious beliefs become political philosophy and lead to legislation that the separation of church from state begins to crumble and the tenets upon which our society was founded are in jeopardy. By imposing religious beliefs upon the entire citizenry the fabric that holds our society together will gradually be torn apart. In the final analysis the state must refrain from interfering with personal freedom. Former Attorney General Ashcroft, an acknowledged Christian Fundamentalist, has opposed Oregon's "Death with Dignity" law. He has directed agents of the Drug Enforcement Administration to act against physicians who prescribe lethal medications to terminally ill Oregon patients. If this is allowed to stand, it will represent an intrusion into the authority of states to regulate their medical practice. Ashcroft's successor, Alberto Gonzales, will contest Oregon's law before the Supreme Court in 2005. Yet the concept of compassion for those with terminal illness considering PAD has expanded across the nation such that there is now a Death with Dignity National Center in Washington, DC.

In 1992 Blendon and co-workers published a large survey that found that 76% of Americans were of the belief that the law should allow the withdrawal of life-sustaining treatment, including food and water, from a terminally ill patient upon request of either the patient or family. With the passage of time opinion polls suggest that the legalization of PAD has substantial public support. In 1982, 68% of Americans supported legally allowing physicians to carry out the terms of a patient's advance directive. By 1991 support had grown to 81%. Indeed, the medical profession is increasingly acknowledging the fact that PAD may have a role in terminal care. Recently the Burlington Free Press published the results of a poll that asked 500 Vermont residents whether they would support or oppose legislation to allow mentally competent adults dying of a terminal disease the choice to request and receive medication to hasten death. The results showed that 77.7% supported it, 17% opposed and 5.3% were not sure.

Sixty percent of surveyed Oregon physicians thought physician-assisted death is ethical and should be legal, and nearly half (46%) would be willing to prescribe a lethal medication. These percentages were slightly lower in a paper by Ganzini and co-workers published five years later. But it was surprising to read that half of the respondents were unsure what to prescribe for this purpose. (Didn't they study pharmacology in medical school?) Those physicians who were not morally opposed to PAD raised practical concerns regarding the writing of a lethal prescription. These included concerns that a patient's family might take legal action if the attempt failed or complications developed; that someone other then the patient might use the prescription; that writing a lethal prescription might violate federal law thus jeopardizing their licenses; or that it would lead to sanctions by hospitals. Many emergency room physicians had similar concerns and felt that safeguards in the Oregon law are inadequate to protect vulnerable patients. A conflict of conscience was also expressed by those who are morally opposed to PAD wondering whether they might be unable to respect the wishes of terminally ill patients. Would they be able to avoid resuscitating patients following a lethal medication? And of course there might be a conflict between the policies of an institution as well as the conscience of the health care provider. In addition, 50% of the physicians were not sure that they could predict that a patient had less then 6 months to live.

Religious faith is a powerful tool, but its opposition to suicide as part of its effort to honor life is flawed when it interferes with the last choice an individual is able to make. The choice of when death should come in a terminal situation belongs to the patient or his family, not the government. Suicide is a matter of individual choice. It has nothing to do with ethics. The present administration seems to delight in playing with our liberties, but when possible, one's death should be one's own choice.

Demographic Characteristics of the 208 Patients Who Died by Physician-Assisted Suicide (PAS) 1998–2004*

Marital Status:
>Married 90 (43%)
>Widowed 47 (23%)
>Divorced 56 (27%)
>Never married 15 (7%)

Underlying Illness:
>Cancer 164 (79%)
>Amyotrophic lateral sclerosis 16 (8%)
>Cardiopulmonary disease 10 (5%)
>Other diseases 18 (8%)

Patients Who Died By PAS:
>Age Median (mean) 69 (25–94)
>Men 108 (52%)
>Women 100 (48%)

Education:
    Less then high school 18 (19%)
    High school graduate 63 (30%)
    Some college 40 (19%)
    College graduate 88 (42%)

Hospice Care:
    Enrolled 178 (86%)
    Declined by patient 28 (13%)
    Unknown 2 (1%)

Lethal Prescriptions:
    Percentage of prescriptions written vs. percentage of pre-scriptions used: 65%

End of Life Concerns Expressed to Physicians:
    Losing autonomy 177 (87%)
    Inability to participate in enjoyable activities 172 (84%)
    Loss of control of bodily functions 121 (59%)
    Burden on family, friends & care givers 74 (36%)
    Loss of dignity 60 (80%)
    Inadequate pain control 45 (22%)
    Financial implications 6 (3%)

* Statistics compiled by The Death with Dignity National Center, 11 Dupont Circle NW, #202, Washington, DC 20036 and the Dept. of Human Services, 800 NE Oregon St., Portland, OR 97232.

Addendum: On January 17, 2006, the United States Supreme Court, by a six-to-three decision adjudicated Oregon's Death with Dignity law in Oregon's favor. By allowing it to stand, it is now the law of the land and other states are free to enact similar laws.

Following service as a Naval officer in World War II, Dr. Tanz completed a Ph.D. in pharmacology. Subsequently he pursued a career of teaching and research in cardiovascular and autonomic pharmacology at several medical schools and also served as visiting professor at the medical schools in South Africa and New Zealand. In 1990 he retired as Professor Emeritus from the Oregon Health Sciences Medical School. Dr. Tanz has authored many scientific articles, textbook chapters and a book. He and his wife of fifty-three years have three children and four grandchildren.

Health, History, and Society

~

Reflections on Our Troubled Times

Donald N. Wysham

Justice

A sense of justice and fair play is a deep-seated, fundamental part of the human psyche. Children quickly develop this sense. People who experience episodes of injustice tend to never forget them. There is a universal feeling among people that justice is a basic right. The Jewish prophets stressed justice—as Micah, who taught "what does the Lord require of you but to do justice" (and to love kindness and walk humbly)[1]; and the magnificent words of Amos: "let justice roll down like waters, and righteousness like an ever-flowing stream."[2]

Ironically, even though the Jewish people have taught the world more about justice, love, and compassion than any other members of the human race, they have been subjected for much of the past two thousand years to greater injustice than should have been their share. This is in part a result of a statement in the New Testament that "the Jews" killed Jesus, and for this act were condemned for all time.[3] Jesus Christ was appreciated and probably considered a hero by the great majority of the Jewish people of his time. However, his teachings were a threat to the Jewish hierarchy, the establishment, and because of this threat he was executed (as was Socrates, also for teachings which threatened the establishment). To blame the entire Jewish people for his execution would be like blaming the English for all time for burning Joan of Arc at the stake, or indicting all white Americans for the murder of Martin Luther King.

In Kashmir, injustice has been the cause of several wars between India and Pakistan, both nuclear powers. The history of the problem dates back to the mid-19th century. Much of what is now northwest India and northern Pakistan comprised the

Sikh Empire, headed by Maharajah Ranjit Singh, with its capital in Lahore. Following some brief wars that were won by the British, the Sikh empire came under the control of Great Britain, which chose to leave the beautiful vale of Kashmir as a "native state" with an Indian ruler, attended by a British political officer—a practice common over much of the rest of India at that time. Almost all of the people living in Kashmir were Muslims. Moreover, their culture and the flora and fauna of Kashmir were related to central Asia, not to India. For example, the Kashmir stag is related to the red deer of Europe, and occurs nowhere else in the Indian subcontinent. Like the maple leaf in Canada, the leaf of the chinar tree (a type of sycamore) is in effect the leaf of the "national" tree of Kashmir, represented in its art and woodwork. The chinar is a common tree in south-western Asia, as in Iran, but not in India.

To create a "native state" of Kashmir, the British needed to appoint as its head a maharajah. There was no local Muslim maharajah suitable for appointment to rule Kashmir, but there were Hindu rajahs ruling other so-called hill states. Hence the British chose to appoint one of these Hindu rajahs as the ruler of Kashmir.

Now fast forward about ninety years to 1947, the year of the partition of India. Maharajah Hari Singh, the Hindu ruler of Kashmir, called for Indian Army troops to be flown into Kashmir to hold it for India, even though predominantly Muslim areas were intended to become part of Pakistan. They had to be flown in because the traditional and natural route in to the mountain-ringed valley of Kashmir was up along the Jhelum River, a tributary of the Indus, through what had become northern Pakistan. Fighting broke out between the Pakistani and Indian armed forces. The problem could have been resolved by a plebiscite. This was suggested by the United Nations, but refused by India, which knew that it could not win. Jawaharlal Nehru, who was the prime minister of India at that time, was born in Kashmir, his family part of the small Hindu minority present there. This probably made it doubly difficult for him to accept the separation of Kashmir from India. It seemed obvious to Pakistan and to the rest of the world that Kashmir should have been part of Pakistan, and the strong sense of injustice on the part of Pakistanis and the residents of Kashmir regarding the present division of Kashmir continues to the present time.

In theory, a solution to the Kashmiri problem should be straightforward. In realpolitik terms, however, it would have to proceed with great delicacy, and a just solution would be difficult to achieve. Ideally, India should allow a plebiscite to occur in the disputed territories of Kashmir. In addition to the options of their joining either India or Pakistan, the Kashmiris should be given a third choice, that of forming an independent state of Kashmir. India could make its acceptance of the results of a plebiscite conditional on an agreement with Pakistan that, in the event that the Kashmiri people opt to join Pakistan or become independent, Kashmir would be readily accessible to Hindus who wish to make a pilgrimage to places which they consider holy, such as the Amarnath Cave. Although this outcome would hurt the national pride of Indians, it would be a much happier result for all concerned than the present impasse. It would be particularly welcome to the residents of Kashmir, partly because they traditionally have benefited from tourism. Once again it would be possible for the rest of us to appreciate the special beauty of the famous Vale—as well as its other delights, such as mountain climbing, trout fishing, etc. Most importantly, a just resolution to the Kashmir problem would significantly reduce the threat of a nuclear war.

Another part of the world where a sense of injustice has been festering for years is the Holy Land—sacred to Jews, Christians, and Muslims. If the question can be addressed objectively, whose land is it, anyway? If we consider its history, most of the Jews living there were removed to Babylon in 597 B.C.E. They were freed from captivity in 538 B.C.E., and the Diaspora (meaning "the scattering") of the Jews occurred. Most of them chose not to return to Palestine but rather to remain in various parts of the Middle East, including Persia. Some migrated further to North Africa or southern Europe, including Spain.[4] Some of the descendants of those who remained in or returned to Palestine migrated away during the period of the domination of the Middle East by the Seleucid Greeks, and many Jews abandoned the region after the destruction of Jerusalem in 70 C.E. and their defeat by the Romans again in 135 C.E. By the time of the Crusades there were relatively few Jews left in Palestine, and, as we all know, the region was occupied by various other Semitic people who were mostly Muslims together with some Christians.

During the Middle Ages, what appears to have been a major factor affecting the future of European Jews was the remarkable development of the kingdom of Khazaria in south-eastern Europe between the sixth and ninth centuries C.E. Geographically, Khazaria surrounded the northern half of the Caspian Sea and extended south to the Caucasus and west to include much of the present Ukraine. By the ninth century C.E., Khazaria was famous for justice and tolerance. Influenced by Jews who were invited to come there from Byzantium and Persia, the king, nobility, and large numbers of the people in Khazaria were converted to Judaism. The descendants of people converted to Judaism in Khazaria and elsewhere in central Europe are known today as the Ashkenazi Jews, who now comprise about 85% of the world's Jews.[5] They are not a Semitic people, but probably are descended from a mixture of the Turkic Khazars and other racial groups living in central Europe during the Middle Ages. (DNA testing can genetically distinguish Ashkenazi from Sephardic Jews.[6] The Sephardic Jews, about fifteen percent of the world's Jewish population, are truly Semitic.)

In a book published in 1956 entitled *Great Ages and Ideas of the Jewish People* is the following statement: "Behind the Zionist movement were, of course, the Jews' ancient yearnings for restoration to the land of their forefathers. In the home, school, and synagogue every growing (Jewish) child received a deep indoctrination in that messianic idea."[7] The accuracy of this statement, including that portion referring to "the land of their forefathers," had no good reason to be challenged in 1956. During the last twenty five years, however, ethnic and genetic studies have shown this portion of the statement to have been a misconception. Ancient Israel was indeed the land of the origin of Judaism, as well as of Christianity and, to a large part, the Muslim faith. However, for most Jews and Christians—and for most Muslims as well—it was not the land of their forefathers. On the other hand, for Sephardic Jews, and for Muslim and Christian Palestinians, the Holy Land certainly was the land of their forefathers, both in the ethnic and religious sense.

Some Zionists and Evangelical Christians ("Christian Zionists") believe that Palestine rightfully belongs to the Jews because God gave it to them very long ago. However, even among Jewish scholars, the stories about Abraham and Moses are considered largely mythical. Moreover, it has been asserted that less than twenty percent of the Jewish citizens of modern Israel are actually practicing Jews. Only the Sephardic Jews can make any claim to having had ancestors who lived in Palestine before the Jews were removed to Babylon in 597 B.C.E. Sephardic Jews comprise about forty percent of the Jews living in Israel (in contrast to their fifteen percent portion of the Jewish Diaspora). If one assumes that twenty percent of Israeli Sephardic Jews believe the stories about Abraham and Moses, it seems that less than ten percent of modern Israelis can claim both from their ancestry and religious conviction that they have a right to occupy any portion of Palestine and dispossess the Palestinians who have been its chief occupants for well over a thousand years.

Does the argument that the Jews have been persecuted and need a homeland, especially after the horror of the Holocaust, justify taking away the homeland of people who have lived there for centuries on end, and to whom portions of the region are also sacred?

The current conflict between heavily armed Israeli military forces and a largely civilian Palestinian population is an instance of gross injustice. The occupation of Palestine by Israelis is somewhat analogous to the violent occupation of predominantly Muslim Bosnia by Orthodox Christian Serbs led by Slobodan Milosevic. That occupation was supposedly justified by the defeat of a Serb army by a Muslim Ottoman Turkish army several hundred years ago. An American Jewish intellectual, Henry Siegman, has carried the analogy further by describing the current policy of Israel as "ethnic cleansing."[8]

In recent years the government of Israel under the leadership of its prime minister, Ariel Sharon, has succeeded in dividing up the West Bank into small circumscribed areas called cantons. It has achieved this with numerous military check points throughout the West Bank, by changes in the highway system of the West Bank, and now by the construction of an enormous serpentine wall—as well as by other repressive measures. The result has been that several million Palestinians are being severely oppressed, and the present situation for Palestinians is similar to a state of siege. Activities that would be normal in one's own country—such as travel for adequate medical care, advanced education, trade, visiting relatives, etc.—have become very difficult or impossible for Palestinians in the cantons.[9] The unemployment rate is extremely high. Many farmers have been unable to reach their fields. Even the aquifer under the West Bank is coming under the control of Israel, so that the water supply of the Palestinians is threatened. The effect of these repressive measures carried out by the Israeli authorities is the creation of onerous conditions for Palestinians living in the West Bank and the Gaza Strip similar to, or even worse than, those of the black population during apartheid in South Africa.

It is not likely that the suppression of the human rights of several million people in this manner can continue indefinitely. For Palestine to function as a viable state requires removal of the various barriers and impediments put in place by the Sharon government in the West Bank. On the other hand, if viable statehood is not granted to the Palestinian population, the final result in the Holy Land will probably be similar to the outcome in South Africa—a single nation, in which Palestinians would be the majority. The objective of Zionists—establishing a "national home" for Jews—would fail.

A solution to the Palestinian–Israeli conflict can only be achieved by the controlling power in the area—the United States. However, for over a hundred years, and increasingly so today, major policy decisions of the United States are determined by small but politically active, well financed political action groups and special interests. For example, our policy toward Cuba is dictated largely by the Cuban lobby, and legislation for gun control by the National Rifle Association through the gun lobby. The resulting legislation may not be in the best interests nor to the liking of the majority of Americans. In the case of Israel, American policy has been influenced for over fifty years by politically active American Jewish Zionists, currently chiefly through AIPAC, the American Israel Public Affairs Committee, now also supported by Christian Zionists. (This is a strange association, since the peculiar fundamentalist theology of the Christian Zionists calls for the ultimate coming of what they call "The Rapture" accompanied by the destruction of Israel and of all of its inhabitants who are not of the Christian Zionist persuasion.) American Zionists have been the source of the power, the engine, for securing support for Israel, which has now exceeded a trillion dollars in military and economic aid over the last half century, paid for by American taxpayers[10]—not counting the aid sent to Israel by private American Jewish organizations. The strong moral support of Israel in the United States has repeatedly prevented intervention by the United Nations in questions involving Israel.

It is claimed that American aid to Israel preserved the only democracy in the Middle East during the Cold War. However, the important ramparts against the spread of Communism were further to the north—Greece and Turkey. The sincerity of our interest in preserving democracy in the region during the Cold War is doubtful since at the same time we helped bring down a representative government in Iran, supported a vicious dictatorship in Iraq, and continued to support other authoritarian Arab regimes in the region. America's primary economic interest in the Middle East was preserving our access to the oil deposits in that region. Our support of Israel angered the Arab countries in which the oil was located, and threatened our economic objectives.

The American Israel Public Affairs Committee is the second most powerful lobby in Congress. AIPAC is so politically powerful in the United States that any of our political leaders opposing its interests does so at considerable risk to his or her political future.[11] In American academia, opposing AIPAC and favoring Palestinians may result in "black-listing" and a threat to academic employment.

AIPAC and related organizations played a major role in the establishment of Israel as a strong Jewish state. However, AIPAC must also accept responsibility for Israel's violations of human rights and international law, and the resulting reactions in Muslim countries to what they consider to be Israel's crimes against humanity. Such reactions have given rise to anti-U.S. terrorist activity, including the horrendous attack on the World Trade Center on September 11, 2001. Such terrorist activity has affected the lives of all Americans, who have supported Israel so generously for the past half-century.

It seems to me that AIPAC and its supporters are the ones in a position to bring about a just solution to the Israeli–Palestinian problem. Most Americans today want such a solution, with justice for both Jews and Palestinians. It is essential for AIPAC to realize that its present policy of unrestricted unilateral support for Israel will ultimately be self-defeating. Were AIPAC instead to strive for justice, and help Israel accept international standards of human rights and international law, a just and peaceful solution to the present strife in the Holy Land could be achieved. Meanwhile, the injustice to the Palestinian people resulting from

Israel's actions is obvious to the rest of the world. It is certainly one of the roots of the terrorism in the Middle East which has changed the lives of all of us for the worse.

Finally, consider the relationship of the United States with Iran. That relationship was a very warm one until 1953, when it was shattered by our unjust actions against the democratically elected government of Iran. In the late nineteenth century, several American colleges were established in the Middle East, including the Presbyterian-related Alborz College in Tehran. This college for men and Sage College, a similar college for women, were almost the only sources of higher education in what was then called Persia. Dr. Samuel Jordan, head of the men's college, introduced soccer to Persia. Soccer has since become the national sport. He and other faculty were highly respected in Persia, and a major avenue in Tehran was named after Dr. Jordan. The first public unveiling of a prominent young Persian Muslim woman occurred at an American school for girls. There were American hospitals offering the only modern medical care in several major cities in Persia. The contributions of Americans in Iran were appreciated by the Iranians.[12] By the end of World War II, America was admired by Iranians, and Americans were welcomed in their fascinating country.

In the 1940s, Mohammad Mossadegh emerged as a progressive Iranian leader. At that time, Iran was a constitutional monarchy ruled by an ineffectual shah but governed by a democratically elected parliament called the Majlis. Mossadegh was appointed prime minister in 1951 over the objections of the shah, and took control of the Iranian government. One of his objectives was to nationalize the Iranian oil fields owned by American and British oil companies. Meanwhile the Cold War was underway. Mossadegh refused to take sides. In 1953, because of concern about Mossadegh's neutrality and the potential loss of control of U.S. and British oil interests in Iran, a coup was organized to bring down the Iranian prime minister. The CIA, working with its British equivalent (MI-6) and with officers of the Iranian army who were loyal to the shah, succeeded in deposing Mossadegh.[13]

The regime which then assumed power in Iran was controlled by conservative elements, though nominally under the rule of the shah. This regime was more compliant toward American and British interests. However, it soon became repressive, with increasing reliance on the use of ruthless secret police, the

Savak, who came to be feared and the regime hated in Iran. This regime was finally replaced in 1979 by a similarly violent fanatical Muslim revolutionary government under the Ayatollah Khomeini. He regarded America as the "Great Satan." In the 1980s, the United States supported Iraq in its war against Iran, even assisting in the supply of chemical and bacteriological weapons. Many thousands of Iranian young men were killed. In 1988, Khomeini ordered the killing of every unrepentant anti-revolutionary political prisoner. It is said that thousands were put to death.[14]

American intervention in 1953 to bring down Mohammad Mossadegh changed the course of Iranian history—and probably very much for the worse. It is reasonable to think that the repressive regime under the shah, the violent revolution of 1979, and possibly even the Iraq–Iran war might not have occurred if Iran had been allowed to continue on its own independent course. In recent years there has been some improvement in U.S.–Iranian relations, but suspicion of our motives and a feeling of injustice remain.

What generalizations and conclusions can be made from these examples of injustice in the world? First, in the last half-century or so, many of those affected by injustice have been Muslims—the people of Kashmir, the Palestinians, and the Iranians. Second, the nation principally responsible for carrying out these injustices is the United States—either directly, or by financing or arming our surrogate, Israel. Third, it is apparent that the sense of injustice felt by some young, intelligent, and well-educated Muslims is so intense that they are willing to sacrifice their lives to seek revenge or to dramatize the desperation felt by their people. One can conclude that a major root of terrorism in the world today is this sense of humiliation and desperation that is felt by people who are affected by injustice. It is no wonder that much of the world is antagonized by the policies of the United States of America.

The response of our country to terrorism has been to fight terrorists wherever we can find them. This policy brings to mind an ancient Greek or Roman myth about a brass warrior. As soon as he was attacked and destroyed, a hundred other brass warriors came up out of the ground.

The leaders of this country do not appear to comprehend the reasons for and the roots of terrorism. Without such understanding, it is not likely that our "war on terrorism" will ever succeed. To find an answer to this problem, we must turn back once again to the Jewish prophets,[15] and apply the Golden Rule to international affairs—namely, to do to other countries and peoples as we would have them do to us. In the words of folk singer Pete Seeger:

> "If we could consider each other . . . a neighbor, a friend, or a brother.
> It could be a wonderful, wonderful world, it could be a wonderful world."

Endnotes

1. Micah 6:8.
2. Amos 5:24.
3. Marcus J.Borg, *The God We Never Knew,* (San Francisco: Harper, 1979) 89, 104.
4. *Microsoft Encarta Encyclopedia Standard 2004*: Babylonian captivity, Diaspora.
5. Kevin Alan Brook, *An Introduction to the History of Khazaria, 1996–2003.* The American Center of Khazar Studies. www.Khazaria.com. (See also "Ashkenazim" in footnote 4 above.)
6. Nicholas Wade, "Geneticists Report Finding Central Asian Link to Levites," *New York Times,* 27 Sept., 2003, A2.
7. Leo W. Schwarz, editor, "Great Ages and Ideas of the Jewish People," NY, *Modern Library,* 1956, 422.
8. Chris Hedges, "Separating Spiritual and Political, He Pays a Price," *New York Times,* 13 June, 2002, A33.
9. Phyllis Bennis, *Understanding the Palestinian-Israel Conflict,* (Lowell, MA:Tari, 2003) 7.
10. David R. Francis, staff writer for the Christian Science Monitor, Economist tallies swell cost of Israel to US, Work & Money: "Economic Scene" Column, 9 Dec. 2002. "Since 1973, Israel has cost the United States about $1.6 trillion. If divided by today's population, that is more than $5,700 per person. This is an estimate by Thomas Stauffer, an economist in Washington."
11. Bennis, Phyllis, *Understanding the Palestinian-Israel Conflict,* (Lowell, MA: Tari, 2003) 23.
12. In 1935 the official name of Persia was changed to Iran, reflecting the Aryan origin of the people.
13. The coup to depose Mossadegh is described in detail in a recent book by Stephen Kinzer, *All the Shah's Men, an American Coup and the Roots of Middle Eastern Terror,* Hoboken: John Wiley & Sons, 2003).
14. Elizabeth Rubin, "The Millimeter Revolution," *New York Times Magazine,* 6 April, 2003, 38–43.
15. Leviticus 19:18; Matthew 22:39.

Terrorism

Terrorism may be defined as the performance of a violent act, often appearing unprovoked, designed to instill fear or terror in a civilian population. There are sporadic episodes of irrational terrorism, with no apparent purpose. A good example was the bombing of the Federal Building in Oklahoma City in 1995.

More commonly acts of terrorism have a specific intent. Usually they are carried out by a relatively impotent group of people who have a specific message and purpose that they cannot convey or achieve by conventional means. A classic example of terrorism for a specific purpose was the assassination of Archduke Francis Ferdinand and his wife in Sarajevo by a Serb nationalist in June 1914.

Two small underground Zionist organizations carried out acts of terrorism against the British in the late 1930s and 1940s in Palestine when it was a British mandate—presumably to encourage the British to leave. These acts included the assassination of a British government official in Palestine, and the bombing of the King David Hotel in Jerusalem in 1946.[1] The latter resulted in the deaths of ninety one persons with many others wounded. It was carried out by a group called the Irgun Zvai Leumi (National Military Organization), commanded by Menachem Begin, who later became a prime minister of Israel. Yitzhak Shamir, who later also attained prominence in an Israeli government, was a member of both the Irgun Zvai Leumi and of the Lohanei Herut Yisrael, also called the Stern Gang, which carried out acts of terrorism against the British and Palestinians. The most blatant act of terrorism for which an Israeli was held responsible was the massacre in 1982 of between 800 and 1500 Palestinians, mostly women, children, and old men, who were living in the "safe" Sabra-Shatila refugee camps in Beirut, Lebanon. Ariel Sharon was in charge of the Israeli military forces in Lebanon at that time, and was later reprimanded by the Israeli government for permitting this massacre to occur. It is said that Sharon hoped that this act of terror would motivate Palestinians to leave their homeland.

Acts of terrorism far greater in magnitude than these were carried out by the armed forces of the United States and Britain in attacks on civilian populations with the expectation that such attacks would shorten World War II and the Vietnam War. On the night of February 14, 1945, a large number of bombers of the

British Air Force dropped fire bombs on Dresden, one of Europe's most beautiful cities. This raid was followed up by an additional air attack by American bombers. The result was the destruction of eighty percent of Dresden and killing an estimated 135,000 people. The fire-bombing of Dresden is considered to have been a particularly vengeful attack since Germany was already at its knees. An "area fire raid" on Tokyo by American B-29 bombers on the night of March 10, 1945, produced a fire storm in which 83,000 people were killed. The atomic bombing of Hiroshima and Nagasaki killed between 100,000 and 240,000 people, almost all civilians. During the Vietnam War napalm was used against civilians. One can never forget the photograph in *Life* magazine of the frantic naked little Vietnamese girl running down a road while being burned by napalm.

The American media have often expressed horror that Palestinian suicide bombers would kill civilians. However, if we include World War II, Vietnam, Cambodia, Angola, Chile, deaths of Iraqi children as a result of sanctions and now of thousands of civilians during the invasion of Iraq, the United States stands out as having directly or indirectly caused the deaths of more innocent civilians than virtually any country in the world's history. It would surely be in the top ten, somewhere behind Genghis Khan, Soviet Russia, and Nazi Germany. We do not have the moral high ground from which to criticize other countries that may cause civilian casualties as they defend their homeland or way of life from foreign aggression.

The attacks on the World Trade Center and on the Pentagon on September 11, 2001, were without doubt episodes of unmitigated horror. The Bush administration has dismissed the significance of these attacks by taking the position that they were caused by terrorists who "can't stand freedom or liberty." It is as though the September 11 attacks are thought to have occurred out of a clear blue sky, for no apparent reason.

The 9/11 attacks were carefully planned and coordinated, and were carried out by intelligent and educated Muslim men who were so dedicated to their cause that they were willing to die for it. To prevent the repetition of this type of terrorist attack it is important to try to understand the mind set of its perpetrators, the reasons for the existence of organizations such as Hezbollah and Al Qaeda, what messages they are aiming to convey, and what they hope to achieve. In other words, we need to know "the reason why."

Osama bin Laden has never fully explained the *raison d'etre* of Al Qaeda. To try to understand his motives and why he is considered a hero by so many young people in the Muslim world, we need to explore the history of the relationship between the West and the Muslim countries of the Middle East.

The Arabs are justifiably proud of their heritage. During the Middle Ages their culture was far more advanced than that of Europe. Even today they recall the vicious and bloody onslaught on their civilization by the Crusaders, whom they probably considered to be crude barbarians. Suspicion of and antipathy toward the West and toward Christianity as a result of the Crusades are considered by some to be among the original roots of conflict in the Middle East today.[2]

The outstanding hero of that period was a leader of Kurdish origin named Saleh-ed-Din, whom the Crusaders called Saladin. He was victorious in war and magnanimous in peace. After taking back Jerusalem, he decreed that Christians and Jews were welcome to come and worship in the holy places in that city.

During and after the first World War and continuing up to the present, there have been a series of events that Arabs, as well as Muslim Iranians, must consider to be examples of arrogant, invasive, insensitive, and even treacherous behavior on the part of western countries—especially Britain and the United States, and more recently by Israel. For fundamentalist Muslims like Osama bin Laden, these events must constitute a bill of particulars which have resulted in pent up frustration, humiliation, and hatred, boiling over into revenge as acts of extreme violence. Some of these events are as follows:

In 1915/1916 the British promised the Arabs independence of their countries after World War I, and therefore the Arabs aided the British in the capture of Palestine from the Ottomans. However, at the same time Britain made secret arrangements to divide and rule the area with its allies. Then in 1917 Britain unilaterally promised to allow the creation in Palestine of a "national home" for Jews by means of the Balfour Declaration. (Recently Jack Straw, the British foreign minister, stated that he feels that the Balfour Declaration was a mistake.)

Over the next twenty years Britain and America, taking advantage of the political weakness of native rule in the Middle East, established ownership and control of oil fields in the region of the Persian Gulf, including areas in southern Iran.

During this same period Zionists envisaged large-scale Jewish immigration into Palestine, which the Palestinians considered to be contrary to promises made to them by the British. Especially during the persecution of Jews in Nazi Germany, many Jews did immigrate into Palestine, nearly 62,000 in 1935. The Arab reaction was intermittent revolt from 1936 to 1939.

In 1947, war broke out between poorly organized Palestinians and the better prepared Jewish military. The Palestinians were defeated. In 1948 the state of Israel was established. President Harry Truman chose to recognize the legitimacy of the state—but not for altruistic reasons. When asked why he had made this decision, he replied that he had many more constituents who were Jews than Arabs.

Upon the declaration that Israel was a state, it was invaded by five Arab armies coming to the aid of the Palestinians. These armies were defeated by Israeli forces and Israel enlarged its territory. In the course of the war, according to a recent report, there were a number of instances of rape of Palestinian women by Israeli soldiers and several massacres of Palestinian civilians by Israeli troops.[3] Some 780,000 Palestinian refugees left their homes. Half did so out of fear or panic. The rest were forced out of their homes and off their land to make room for Jewish immigrants. About 150,000 embittered Palestinian refugees entered Lebanon, where the population was mostly Arab.

In 1953, in Iran, the democratically elected prime minister, Mohammad Mossadegh, was overthrown, largely by covert actions of agents of the CIA and its British equivalent.[4] A despotic regime came to power in Iran—one that was compliant with British and American oil interests.

In 1967 a pre-emptive war initiated by Israel against its Arab enemies, the so-called Six-Day War. The Arab forces were soundly defeated. As a result another wave of Palestinian refugees entered Lebanon, where fighting occurred between members of the Palestine Liberation Organization and various Lebanese factions.

In 1979 the Muslim revolutionary government was established in Iran under Ayatollah Khomeini, who branded the United States "The Great Satan."

Between 1980 and 1988 the Iran–Iraq war occurred. In this conflict, the United States took the side of Iraq, and together with some European countries supplied Iraq with weapons for chemical and bacteriological warfare. Many Iranian troops were killed or permanently disabled by the Iraqi use of poison gas (as were civilian Kurds). Our support of Saddam Hussein was resented by Iran and also probably by Osama bin Laden who, as a conservative Muslim, opposed Saddam's secular government in a Muslim country.

To pacify the Palestinians and to punish Lebanon for hosting them, Israel launched a full-scale invasion of Lebanon in June, 1982. Nearly 18,000 Lebanese, in addition to many Palestinians and (Arab) Syrians, were killed in the Israeli invasion. It was at this time that the civilian Palestinian refugees in the Sabra-Shatila refugee camps in Beirut were massacred. (In October 1983 more than 300 U.S. and French troops were killed in their barracks in Beirut by a truck bomb.)

Meanwhile over a million Palestinian Arab refugees were living in the Gaza Strip, which amounts to a massive refugee camp. In the Strip there is a great deal of poverty, unemployment, poor sanitary conditions, poor health—especially of the children—despair, and festering anger directed toward Israel.

Muslims regarded the Persian Gulf War in 1991 as motivated largely by the desire to secure access to the oil fields of Kuwait for the West. It is unlikely that the war would have occurred if in 1990 Saddam Hussein's army had invaded empty desert.

The presence of American armed forces residing in Saudi Arabia, regarded as sacred territory by fundamentalist Muslims, has been cited by Al Qaeda as one reason for its anger with this country.

The United States continues to support Israel in its bitter confrontation with those Palestinians still residing in the Gaza Strip or the West Bank, where sophisticated American heavy weapons, such as attack helicopters, are used against lightly armed Palestinians. It is claimed that, in addition to giving Israel over a trillion dollars in support over the past fifty years, the United States has for years paid several billion dollars per year to Egypt to refrain from anti-Israeli activities.[5] The brutal suppression of a civilian Palestinian population by our surrogates, the Israeli Army, armed with American heavy weapons, is a major blot on the history of civilization. It continues to cause hatred for Israel and the United States throughout the Muslim world. Meanwhile Israel has refused to honor over sixty-nine United Nations' resolutions and international agreements. The

United States has blocked or vetoed over twenty UN resolutions condemning Israel, including a recent resolution criticizing Israel for the murder of a Red Cross worker in his office.

In summary, we Americans will have to come to realize that terror is terror, and horror is horror, whether we do it to others, have it done to others by our surrogates or as the result of our policies or activities, or whether they do it to us. Human life is no more valuable in the United States than in Vietnam, Iraq, or the Gaza Strip. Although it is horrible to jump out of a burning building in New York City, it is perhaps worse to be tortured and then dropped into the Pacific, as the result of our arranging the ousting of Allende and supporting Pinochet. We have so far escaped most of the horror in the world, and have suffered a tiny fraction of the terror our policies have caused people in other countries.

We must accept as a fact that our policies and actions over the last century in the Middle East, the Far East, and Latin America, and more recently the actions of our surrogate, Israel, are to blame for much of the hatred felt for us in the Middle East and elsewhere in the world. Until we look into a mirror and see ourselves as others see us, terrorism—by both sides—will in all likelihood continue.

Endnotes

1. This together with most other facts and figures in this essay were either confirmed by or derived from the Microsoft Encarta, 2004.
2. Karen Armstrong, *Holy War: The Crusades and their Impact on Today's World,* New York: Anchor Books, 2001 xiv.
3. Ari Shavit, Survival of the fittest, an interview with Benny Morris. www.palestineremembered.com/Acre/Articles/Story117.html. Posted on 11 Jan. 2004.
4. Stephen Kinzer, *All the Shah's Men: An American Coup and the Roots of Middle East Terror,* Hoboken, John Wiley & Sons, 2003.
5. David R. Francis, Work and Money: "Economic Scene" Column, 9 Dec. 2002.

Iraq

Note: The following essay was written in November 2003, and reflects the thinking of those many Americans who were opposed to a pre-emptive military strike against Iraq.

When the people of any country perceive that they are threatened by a possible external attack, they close ranks and rally around the flag. This axiom was apparently in the mind of Karl Rove, President George W. Bush's political manager. In his inaugural speech the President implied that this country was threatened by an "axis of evil" consisting of Iran, Iraq, and North Korea. The psychology of fear has been used repeatedly ever since as a political tool by the Bush administration.

In his speech to the Republican National Committee in January, 2002, Karl Rove announced that the "war on terror" would be a key factor leading to victory for the Republican party in the mid-term elections later that year. Meanwhile the surge in popularity of the Bush administration following 9/11 had begun to subside, possibly because Osama Bin Laden had not been captured. During the rest of 2002, a propaganda blitz was organized by the Bush administration to create the belief in the minds of most Americans that Saddam Hussein, an evil tyrant, was partly responsible for 9/11, that he possessed "weapons of mass destruction" (WMD), and his regime posed a real and imminent threat to this country—even by the potential use of nuclear weapons. The threat of a "mushroom cloud" was specifically described by a senior member of the administration. A cabal including Karl Rove, Paul Wolfowitz, Dick Cheney, and Donald Rumsfeld pushed for a pre-emptive military strike against Iraq in pursuit of the "war on terror." By the fall of 2002 over 70% of the American people believed that Saddam Hussein was a major threat to this country, and that he was partly responsible for 9/11. The Bush administration won the November mid-term election, giving the administration control over both branches of the Congress. The Bush team was now in position to carry out its agenda.

Consider the claim that Iraq was harboring weapons of mass destruction (WMD). To make an issue of this in August, 2002, was suspicious for several reasons. First, Saddam Hussein had not made a significantly provocative move for years. Moreover, the CIA announced that it had no recent information about Iraq's weapons—and had not had such information for about five years. Then why this sudden concern, out of a clear blue sky, so to speak? The validity of the WMD claim became more suspect as the UN team failed to find any such weapons in Iraq.

What about the claim of the Bush administration that Iraq was partly responsible for 9/11, and that therefore the "war against terror" should include a pre-emptive attack on Iraq? It was well known that Osama and Saddam Hussein were enemies—Osama opposed the secularization of a Muslim state as had happened in Iraq. Also, it appeared that there were a number of Al Qaeda operatives in Germany and in the United States, but little or no connection could be established between Al Qaeda and Iraq—in contrast to Saudi Arabia, where there was the obvious connection to 9/11. Thus it was apparent that this claim was false, and merely part of the propaganda blitz to frighten the American people—and it worked! Most Americans came to believe that Al Qaeda had a connection with Iraq, that Saddam Hussein was partly responsible for 9/11, and that Iraq was hiding WMD. They rallied around the flag, and the Republicans won the mid-term election.

The Bush administration also gave as a reason for pre-emptive war against Iraq the fact that Saddam Hussein has been an evil dictator, and it would be best to replace his regime with a democracy which would serve as a model and inspiration for the Middle East. This rationale is probably not only untrue, but also hypocritical. There have been many evil dictators in the past, such as Stalin, Idi Amin, and Pinochet, but the United States has never been in the business of pre-emptively attacking them. In fact, for much of the twentieth century, and especially during the Cold War, the United States. had no hesitation in doing just the opposite by conniving to bring down representative governments, such as those of Iran and Chile, and seeing them replaced with repressive dictatorial regimes. Moreover, if Iraq were to be a democracy, the first government elected would probably be a strongly anti-American theocratic regime such as that in Iran.

In the case of Chile, Salvador Allende was elected president in 1970. He was a socialist, and planned the nationalization of some American-owned companies. President Richard Nixon objected to Allende because of his leftist leanings and his plans to nationalize U.S. companies. The CIA gave ten million dollars covertly to aid Allende's opponents. However, the general who was the chief of staff of Chile's army remained loyal to Allende. According to a segment in the CBS program "60 Minutes," President Nixon conferred with his Secretary of State, Henry Kissinger, who concurred that it would be necessary to arrange the removal of this general if a coup were to succeed. The CIA was instructed to kidnap the general, who resisted and was killed. On Sept. 11, 1973, Allende was overthrown by a violent military coup, and died of bullet wounds. General Augusto Pinochet led a repressive military dictatorship which lasted for sixteen years, and was accompanied by the murder or disappearance of thousands of Pinochet's opponents, including many civilians.

Thus it appears that the Bush administration has used the "Big Lie" as a propaganda tool, as did the Nazi government of Germany in the 1930s. This would not have been the first time for the United States. The U.S. battleship Maine exploded and sank in Havana harbor in 1898 with heavy loss of life, and the government allowed the assumption to persist that it was sabotaged by the Spanish. "Remember the Maine" rang out as a battle cry to arouse public support for the war which followed, even though an investigation showed that there had been a spontaneous coal fire causing an explosion in the ship's boilers. Again in 1964, President Lyndon Johnson used a false story of an attack by the North Vietnamese against American warships in the Gulf of Tonkin to persuade Congress and the U.S. public to accept escalating the war against North Vietnam.

So what were the probable real reasons for the invasion of Iraq in 2003? The first has already been described—namely, the need to find a new threat to galvanize the American public and win the mid-term election of 2002. Second, there may well have been an ego factor in the case of the President, who probably wanted to finish what his father had begun in the Persian Gulf War ("Desert Storm") a dozen years previously. Perhaps George W. Bush had not read his father's book warning of the combination of hornet's nest and quagmire that would most likely result from an American attempt to replace Saddam Hussein. The elder Bush wrote, presciently:

> Trying to eliminate Saddam . . . would have incurred incalculable human and political costs . . . We would have been forced to occupy Baghdad and, in effect, rule Iraq. . . . there was no viable 'exit strategy' we could see . . . Had we gone the invasion route, the United States could conceivably still be an occupying power in a bitterly hostile land. (George Bush and Brent Scowcroft, *A World Transformed,* NY, Alfred A. Knopf, Inc., 1998, 489.)

It is also probable that his own impulse to eliminate Saddam made it easy for President George W. Bush to go along with what were reported to have been additional motives of the above mentioned cabal of Rove et al. The rationale of this group is reported to have included the belief that the removal of Saddam Hussein would help protect Israel, and the desire to maintain a degree of control over the supply of oil from the Middle East. (Ironically, aiding and protecting Israel and ensuring oil supplies have been the inherently conflicting policies of the U.S. government in the Middle East for more than fifty years.)

Consider the moral and ethical aspects of the decision to attack Iraq if the chief motives were the 2002 mid-term election, the President's ego, maintaining control over another country's oil reserves, and protecting Israel—a country accused of ethnic cleansing and led by Ariel Sharon, who has been charged of being a war criminal by Belgium for his part in the 1982 massacre in Lebanon of Palestinian refugees. Imagine trying to justify to the American people and to the rest of the world the deaths of hundreds of American soldiers, thousands of Iraqis, enormous destruction of the infrastructure of a country, and hundreds of billions of dollars in expense, for these reasons. Thus it was essential to persuade the American public of acceptable reasons, namely a real and immediate threat from WMD, pursuing Al Qaeda and the war on terrorism, and establishing democracy while getting rid of a monster for the Iraqi people.

To better understand the moral problem, think of the world in terms of a global village in which you object to the way a neighbor runs his affairs, and whose property you envy. Therefore you decide to attack him, kill many members of his family and retainers, destroy his house, and assume control over his property. You would be committing murder, as well as other criminal acts. A war that is inadequately justified is mass murder, and its perpetrators are war criminals.

Looking back over U.S. history, it is not hard to find instances of wars for which there was little justification, such as the war with Mexico in 1846, the Spanish–American War, and several little wars in Central America and the Caribbean. There are also the many surreptitious interventions, without the approval of Congress, such as facilitating the overthrow of the Allende government in Chile or the Mossadegh government in Iran, both of which resulted in enormous numbers of deaths, disappearances, instances of torture, and so forth. Nor is this the first time that our government has carried on with a war partly for domestic political reasons. There was a point in the Vietnam War when President Johnson and his adviser, Henry Kissinger, conferred about the fact that they knew that the war could not be won, but to publicly admit and announce that fact would be politically damaging. They therefore decided to continue the war, resulting in the deaths of thousands more U.S. troops and untold thousands of Vietnamese, Laotians, and Cambodians.

Epilogue (November 2005): In the two years that have elapsed since this essay was composed, most of the suspicions and dire predictions of those who protested the pre-emptive Iraq war have been confirmed by events in Iraq. The strategy used by Karl Rove and the rest of the pro-war cabal, that of using the Big Lie to mislead the American people regarding the *raisons d'etre* for the Iraq war, was not only successful in winning the mid-term national elections of 2002, but the American public continued to believe these deceits until November 2004, when over seventy percent of Americans still believed that Saddam Hussein was in league with Al Qaeda and partly responsible for the 9/11 attacks on the United States. The result was that President George W. Bush was re-elected for another term. Thus, partly by the use of the Big Lie, and since gaining control of both houses of the Congress in 2002, the Republican administration won six uninterrupted years to carry out its domestic agenda.

The cost of this victory, however, has been enormous. In addition to many billions of war-related expenses, the Bush administration has lost the confidence of the American people, and the United States has lost respect and prestige in the rest of the world. Also, it is difficult to avoid the conclusion that, partly for their personal political gain, the leaders of this Bush administration have been willing to sacrifice the lives and limbs of thousands of young men and women in the U.S. armed forces, as well as to kill or seriously injure tens of thousands of innocent Iraqi civilians. In this author's opinion, these leaders appear to have been guilty of the "high crimes and misdemeanors" mentioned in the Constitution of the United States of America.

How is it that we Americans, who individually are such friendly, helpful, exceptionally church-going, nice people, come to this time in our history when our government is considered by most of the world to be probably the greatest threat to world peace? That is part of the subject of the next essay.

America

What is wrong with America? Why do we do such a poor job of picking our political leaders? Why do so many people in the world today hate us? Why do we sometimes wish that we live in New Zealand or Canada?

The answers to some of these questions are dealt with in two fairly recent books. Robert D. Putnam, the author of *Bowling Alone*[1] reports and discusses the disintegration of American society that has occurred over the past fifty years or so. We used to join organizations—such as bowling leagues, the P.T.A., the League of Women Voters, and service clubs. We now tend to live our own individual lives.

The second book, *Habits of the Heart,*[2] is a report of a sociological study of American society funded by the Ford and Rockefeller Foundations and the National Endowment for the Humanities. The authors point out that Americans are united by one core belief: "that economic success or misfortune is the individual's responsibility, and his or hers alone . . . This common American belief is shared by the population of no other industrial nation, either in Europe or East Asia."[3] The authors relate this belief, with reference to Alexis de Tocqueville,[4] to American individualism, which values independence and self-reliance above all else. They point out that our individualism stimulates great energy to achieve, but provides little nurturing of moral development. Inspired by de Tocqueville, they argue that "individualism has been sustainable in the United States only because it has been supported and checked by other, more generous moral understandings. . . . Individualism alone does not allow persons to understand certain basic realities of their lives, especially interdependence with others."[5] The nation's founders were immersed in the Biblical tradition, with the result that they insisted "that the American experiment is a project of common moral purpose, one which places upon citizens a responsibility for the welfare of their fellows and for the common good."[6]

Radical individualism alienates people from a sense of commitment, of community, and of citizenship. The resulting crisis in civic participation which has resulted, especially in the last decade or so, threatens the "confident sense of selfhood that comes from membership in a society in which we believe, where we both trust and feel trusted, and to which we feel we securely belong."[7] In America today there has been an enormous and widening gulf between the very rich and the rest of society, exaggerated by our current income tax structure. This has resulted in the formation of a powerful elite who have a "loss of civic consciousness, of a sense of obligation to the rest of society, which leads to a secession from society into guarded, gated residential enclaves and ultra-modern offices, etc."[8] This elite has a "predatory attitude toward the rest of society . . . [and a] willingness to pursue its own interests without regard to any one else."[9] The authors feel "that the extreme position of the United States compared to other countries in matters such as income inequality and the attack on public provision is due in important part to the culture of individualism, with its inability to understand the capacities and responsibilities of government."[10]

These authors quote a sermon delivered by John Winthrop to the Massachusetts Bay colonists in 1630, as follows: "If we pursue our pleasures and profits we will surely perish in this good land."[11] In today's society, however, we tend to forget our obligations of solidarity and community, to harden our hearts and look out only for ourselves. Referring to Lincoln's "House Divided" speech, the authors express the belief that the class difference of today is wrong, indicating that "a house divided against itself cannot stand."[12] They point out that a characteristic of most of the great religions and philosophies of mankind is the idea of turning away from preoccupation with self and toward some larger identity,[13] with a realization that individuals live in a society that has a common good beyond the sum of individual goods.[14] John Winthrop, paraphrasing the Apostle Paul, tells us that "we must be willing to abridge ourselves of our superfluities, for the supply of others' necessities . . . we must delight in each other, make others' conditions our own, rejoice together, mourn together, labor and suffer together, always before our eyes . . . our Community as members of the same Body."[15]

In contemporary America where there is a progressively greater gulf in incomes and the existence of a body of the super-rich, more than ever before vast amounts of money are available with which to influence politics. There is a pressing need for more campaign reform. The recently enacted McCain–Feingold reform bill is a move in the right direction, but further restrictions are needed to prevent the ultra-wealthy from, in effect, purchasing candidates of their choosing.

Another important and related problem in our form of democracy is lobbying. This practice derives its legitimacy from Article One of the First Amendment to the United States Constitution, which guarantees people the right to petition their government. The presumption that it also has led to extensive corruption for many years is suggested by the remark of Mark Twain over a century ago, to the effect that we have the best government (or Congress) that money can buy. Another reference to the debasing effect of lobbies on democracy comes from Winston Churchill in 1904. He felt that protective tariffs would lead to "the Americanization of English politics," referring to the corrupting effect of lobbies whereby the industrial interests with the "longest purses and least scruples would get the highest duties."[16] It may be surprising to learn that lobbyists are permitted to attend committee meetings in Congress, where they presumably are allowed to express their views, thus directly influencing committee decisions.

The effectiveness of the lobby for Israel (AIPAC) demonstrates the remarkable strength of lobbies in our government. For many years it has exerted a large measure of influence over the Middle East policy of this country. As mentioned previously in these essays, AIPAC has persuaded our government to spend, directly or indirectly, approximately a trillion of U.S. taxpayer dollars in support of Israel. The Cuban lobby in Miami and the lobby of the National Rifle Association have both managed to influence our laws and policies in ways that far exceed the demographic weight of their constituents. The consequences of these lobbying efforts seem to many to be irrational and ultimately harmful to the national interest. Largely as a result of the power and influence of lobbies, we do not have a democracy in the Lincolnian sense. Rather we have a government of the people by special interests for the benefit of special interests. The power of lobbies is exaggerated by the financial gulf between the super-rich and the rest of us, which gulf in turn is widened by our current tax laws, including phasing out of the inheritance tax.

We look down on other countries of the world because of their corrupt politics and demean some with the appellation of "banana republic," but in fact the outcome of our national elections is no doubt determined in part by money, and the effect of lobbying is essentially the same as what we call "bribery" overseas. We are reluctant to use that word when describing our own political scene. It is very likely that we would have much finer types of men and women entering politics today—the George Washingtons, Abraham Lincolns, and George C. Marshalls of our day and their female equivalents—were it not necessary for them to raise huge amounts of money for presidential election or, at the level of Congress, to enter an atmosphere of compromised integrity created by lobbying.

Legislation to limit the power of lobbies could surely be achieved without significantly limiting the right of people to petition their government. However, the Congress will have great difficulty achieving this type of reform, controlled as it is by lobbies. Strong presidential leadership might be able to accomplish this result.

Another major impediment to making ours a true democracy, a government by the people, is our attitude toward our Constitution as though it were sacrosanct, or engraved in stone. As a result, we are very reluctant to bring about changes in our electoral system which would make it more appropriate for America today.

The founders of our country were indeed very high-minded, intelligent, educated, and public-spirited gentlemen, but they certainly could not foresee the future in all of its aspects. Moreover, the United States of America, created from a federation of thirteen colonies in the 1780s, was very different from the present United States of America. In the original states there was not as great variance as today in their population. Communication was very slow. The population of each state was relatively stable—people did not move as much from state to state then as they do today. Each state demanded roughly equal representation in the national senate and in the election of a president of the United States before it would agree to ratify the Constitution. Finally, the states were divided by the institution of slavery, which was supported by about half of the states at that time. The slave states insisted on having political power equal to that of the non-slave states.

In the United States today, there is not as much difference in the character and requirements of the states as there was two hundred years ago. States rights is not as much of an issue now as it once was. People do not feel the same sense of devotion and identity with their home state as they once did. as they move freely from state to state. It no longer makes sense for Rhode Island, with a population of one million people, to have the same representation in the United States Senate as New York

State, with a population of nineteen million. Relatively speaking, the citizens of New York State are partially disenfranchised in the U. S. Senate, where many crucial decisions are made. With some thought it should not be difficult to devise a much more equitable system for representation in the United States Senate. For example, there could be a minimum of one or two senators for states with populations up to five million people, with another senator to represent each additional five million of population. Thus Rhode Island would have one or two senators, California eight, and New York State five. Such a system could preserve the present practice of having each senator represent the whole state, and being elected for a six year term, thus differentiating it from the election for the U.S. House of Representatives.

The Electoral College is another anachronism. The electors choose the president and the vice president of the United States. Each state is entitled to a number of electors equal to the total of the senators and representatives which it sends to the United States Congress. With the exception of the states of Maine and Nebraska, which allow their electoral votes to be split, all of the electors in each of the other states vote as a unit, the so called "winner-take-all" system. Thus, for example, if in the state of California ten million people vote for one candidate for president and just under ten million for another, all of California's fifty five electoral votes will go to the first candidate—theoretically even if the difference were just one vote. This system has resulted in a candidate winning the presidency even though he may have received fewer popular votes than his opponent—as in the case of the election in the year 2000 when George W. Bush defeated Al Gore. Clearly this system occasionally prevents the candidate who is the popular choice from winning the presidency. Many of its critics feel that the Electoral College system should be abolished and replaced by direct popular election.[17]

True democracy in this country is also subverted by another aspect of our system for electing a president. Often there are more than two candidates running for president, with candidates representing parties additional to the standard two parties. This occasionally results in a candidate for president being elected by receiving a plurality of votes, even though it is apparent that a majority of the population would not choose that candidate in a run-off presidential election, as is held in other countries. This occurred in 1912 when Theodore Roosevelt organized a third party, the Progressive ("Bull Moose") Party, thus splitting the Republican vote. More recently, in the 2000 election, those who . voted for Ralph Nader would mostly likely have, in a run-off election, voted for the other environmentally friendly candidate, Al Gore, who would then have won the presidency. It is not difficult to understand that, in the 1780s, a run-off election would have been very awkward, but today conditions are different. With some effort by interested parties, elections could be electronic, and a run-off election need not take much more than a few days time to be accomplished.

There is a great deal of voter apathy in America. This would be a cause of concern in any democracy, but in the United States, the most powerful nation in the world today, it is not only of concern, but it is dangerous for the rest of the world. The causes of voter apathy are no doubt multiple, but among them are the various imperfections in American democracy discussed above—namely, the belief that "big money" determines the outcome of elections, impatience with chronic corruption in Washington, the relative absence of outstanding candidates for office, the controlling role of special interests and lobbies in our government, and our outdated and cumbersome election design and voting techniques. If a person feels disenfranchised and believes that his or her voting is ineffectual, there will surely be a tendency to not vote. The answer is not for us to move to Canada or New Zealand, but rather to strive to achieve better executive leadership in Washington, DC, whereby the failures in our democracy may ultimately be corrected.

Endotes

1. Robert D. Putnam, *Bowling Alone: the Collapse and Revival of American Community,* NY, Simon and Shuster, 2000
2. Robert N. Bellah, Richard Madsen, William M. Sullivan, Ann Swidler and Steven M. Tipton, *Habits of the Heart: Individualism and Commitment in American Life,* Berkeley: University of California Press, 1996
3. Ibid, viii.
4. Alexis de Tocqueville was a prominent Frenchman who traveled extensively in America in the 1830s, studying our political system. The results of his studies were published in volumes entitled *Democracy in America,* one of the earliest and most profound studies of American life.
5. Ibid, ix.

6. Ibid.
7. Ibid, xi.
8. Ibid, xii.
9. Ibid.
10. Ibid, xviii.
11. Ibid, xxxv.
12. Mark 3:25.
13. Robert N. Bellah, et al., xxxi.
14. Ibid, xxxiv.
15. Ibid, xxv.
16. Roy Jenkins, Churchill, New York, Farrar, Straus and Giraux, 2001, 85
17. *Microsoft Encarta Encyclopedia Standard 2004*: Electoral College

Energy

Our need for energy, especially oil, has dictated part of our foreign policy for at least half a century. It is most likely one of the causes of our current impasse in Iraq. Also, our dependence on energy from fossil fuels is certainly one of the chief causes of global warming, which is changing life on this planet, and will be a progressively greater threat to life as we know it unless we can come up with a suitable alternative.

Renewable energy sources, such as the sun and wind, are appealing since they will not add to global warming, but they are unlikely to be able to supply a large proportion of our energy needs without becoming an ecological problem in themselves. Wind farms are a blight on the landscape, and the same would be true of square miles of solar energy panels. There should be little objection to placing solar panels on every roof in the sun-belt of this country, but this would surely meet only part of our needs. Fuel cells may one day be useful for cars, but just now we need an alternative source of power other than fossil fuels for industries and for our cities, as well as for transportation.

A number of European countries and Japan are turning more to nuclear energy as their answer to this problem. We in the United States have been reluctant to expand the use and development of nuclear power as a major source of energy. We have been concerned about the safe disposal of nuclear waste. We have also been concerned about the threat to public safety of nuclear power plants, especially after the Chernobyl disaster.

With regard to the first concern, there does appear to be a reasonable solution. Geologists have shown that North America has been in approximately its present form for about 100 million years. If one were to bore a shaft down almost anywhere in North America to a point below sea level, and then create a series of radiating side tunnels, one would have a storage area for nuclear waste where it would almost certainly stay in place for millions of years, and would be no ecological threat.

Certainly nuclear power plants would best be placed at some distance from population centers. Our nuclear scientists have presumably learned from past disasters how to improve the structural safety of such plants.

Deriving most of our power from nuclear energy would make us independent of Middle Eastern oil. It would markedly simplify our foreign policy, while helping to reverse or at least stabilize damage to the ozone layer and help prevent global warming. What we need is strong national leadership with an open mind and vision for the future.

Dr. Wysham was born in Tehran, Persia, in 1928, the son of American Presbyterian missionaries. During his medical career he was for ten years on the faculty of the Christian Medical College, Ludhiana, in Punjab, India, and served for several years as Associate Professor of Medicine. He subsequently was on the clinical teaching staff of the Oregon Health Science University, Portland, Oregon. His medical specialty was cardiology. He has been a lifelong student of history.

A Futurist Looks at Societal Issues

Donald B. Louria

Our educational system is dysfunctional in one aspect that is crucial to how our society functions and whether it will thrive. We are not teaching students how to think critically, and we are not adequately preparing them for long-term commitment to solving major societal problems. Apparently mesmerized by the extraordinary advances in communications technologies and the capacity to gather information, we have hoodwinked ourselves into the assumption that information is equivalent to understanding. They are not identical. Information may be required to develop understanding, but understanding is a far broader concept. Similarly, understanding by itself does not equal critical thinking, though it is usually an essential component. I and my colleagues propose a change in our educational approach that could make a huge difference; we believe we should include, as an intrinsic part of the curriculum, attempts to instill in students what we have called societally connected thinking, a form of critical thinking that blends interdisciplinary learning with systems thinking. This has not been a significant component of the educational process; instead, for the last four decades, our educational efforts have, in large part, focused on incorporation of technological advances. As a consequence, we now have generations of decision makers at local, state, national, or international levels who, in the aggregate, are inadequately trained to solve or even ameliorate major problems that threaten the future of our society. This may help explain the terrible mess the current administration has made in regard to international and national policies.

Unless we imbue our students at all educational levels with the need to think in a societally connected way, we will continue to develop decision makers who are unable to cope with the increasing complexity of the world, and a public that is not committed to participate in seeking solutions to major problems. This could lead to a societal catastrophe.

There are three interrelated components of societally connected thinking. These are:

1. Obligatory interdisciplinary courses: At every educational level—junior high school, high school, college—the curriculum should include mandatory interdisciplinary courses that cover the current major problems facing society at local, state, national, and international levels, as well as the critical problems we are likely to face in future years, decades, and centuries.

2. Systems (non-linear) thinking: Students, including medical and other graduate students, must be taught to think about complex problems in a manner that is comprehensive, integrated, and holistic, and that uses the principles of systems thinking. That is the bedrock of our proposal. We, as a society, including our politicians and leaders, usually address complex problems in a simplistic fashion with comfortably linear approaches, even though these problems require a much broader, systems approach. It has been said that there are often simple solutions that can be found for complex problems, but they are usually wrong.

3. Commitment to problem solving: Our educational system must conscientiously and deliberately seek to instill in students a long-term, part-time, or even full-time, commitment to addressing major societal problems and a commitment to lifelong learning. Active individual participation in problem solving can be at local, state, national, or international levels.

In decades past, we taught civics, making the assumption it would engender commitment. It infrequently did. Currently, some schools require participation in community projects, but this, too, is not likely to result in lifetime dedication to solving or ameliorating critical societal problems unless the concept of commitment is vigorously nurtured throughout students' educational experience.

One problem is that many young people will be concerned that, as individuals, they can have no significant impact on major societal problems. As Sidney Smith, a 19th century British clergyman, noted (quotation slightly modified), "No man or woman makes a greater mistake than to do nothing because he or she can only do a little." To cope with those concerns, attempts at instilling commitment must be accompanied by specific involvement that is rewarding enough to persuade students they can indeed make a difference.

Two health-related examples will illustrate the usefulness of the systems approach; the problems of emerging and re-emerging infections and of drug use.

The Problem of Emerging and Re-Emerging Infections: Emerging infections are those that are either new or occur in a new geographic area. Re-emerging infections are those that have been dormant for a prolonged period and then reappear. HIV/AIDS is the prototype of a ferocious emerging infection epidemic. Diphtheria in the 1990s in Russia and ex-Soviet Union countries is an example of an infection that re-emerged, in large part because of public health infrastructure breakdown. Such infections can arise spontaneously or be deliberately created (biologic terrorism or warfare). In reacting to the concerns about such epidemics, the public health and scientific communities have focused on better surveillance to detect such epidemics early, rapid laboratory diagnosis, and prompt intervention.

That is a perfectly reasonable approach, but it is essentially linear and simplistic. Although surveillance and prompt diagnosis are necessary, coping with and preventing these ferocious epidemics requires a much more comprehensive, systems approach. I am convinced that the most effective way to control the frequency and severity of emerging infection epidemics is to do something about the major societal variables that provide the milieu in which emerging infections arise and thrive. The two superordinating determinants are population growth and global warming. Others include massive urbanization with disease-promoting slums, increase in the number of people living in poverty, larger numbers of refugees, wars, an aging population, the search for energy, malnutrition, increased international travel, and certain human behaviors. I will expand a bit on the two major determinants: population size and global warming.

Population growth: Modern civilization dates from approximately 10,000 B.C. It took almost that entire span for the planetary population to reach one billion persons. Once that milestone was achieved (in 1830), the population express gathered steam. It required only 100 years for world population to double to two billion, and seventy more years to reach six billion. Fertility rates are falling so that some developed countries are at zero population growth, but overall world population is growing at a rate of 1.2 percent per annum, with a projected population doubling time of 58 years. It seems almost certain there will be 8 billion people on the planet by the year 2040, with a likely eventual planetary population of between nine and eleven billion people.

Global Climate Change: The climatological event most likely to affect infectious diseases is global warming. The evidence for global warming is now convincing. It is likely that, by the end of this century, the planet will be 1.5°C to 4°C warmer. At least one-half the greenhouse gas burden is due to carbon dioxide. Methane (10 to 20 percent), chlorofluorocarbons (10 to 20 percent), and nitrogen oxides (4 to 7 percent) are the other principal greenhouse gases. More than 25 billion tons of carbon dioxide are released yearly into the environment. Atmospheric carbon dioxide concentrations have risen 30 percent in the last two centuries; the current concentration of 375 parts per million may increase by an additional 60 percent by the end of the twenty-first century.

Unless vigorous action is taken, greenhouse gas emissions will inevitably increase as world population grows. The warming will result in winners and losers. Some geographic areas will be more productive; others will suffer from severe floods or drought, both guaranteed to increase the number and flow of refugees. Some 500 million people now live at or near sea level. Global warming and the resultant flooding that will likely follow will displace tens of millions, perhaps hundreds of millions, of these sea level inhabitants. Seawater incursions will destroy wetlands and contaminate fresh water supplies.

At higher temperatures, some disease-carrying mosquitoes tend to be more active, eat more voraciously, and bite more frequently. Additionally, they have more rapid reproductive cycles and the time required for development of infectious agents, such as malaria, in the mosquito is lessened. Mosquitoes that at present find higher elevations cold and inhospitable will be able to thrive in previously mosquito-free areas that have become warmer. This, in turn, will introduce mosquito-borne diseases, such as malaria and dengue, to previously unexposed areas.

Malaria, dengue, and schistosomiasis lead the list of infections likely to increase as a consequence of global warming. Malaria is perhaps the most feared disease on the planet. There are an estimated 300 to 500 million people affected each year with one to three million deaths. Only tuberculosis rivals malaria in the number of deaths. Global warming could markedly increase the number of cases. Dengue is a viral disease transmitted by mosquitoes that affects 100 million persons yearly. In most persons, it causes fever, chills, and severe muscle aches, with recovery in a period of several days to several weeks. However, in those who have had previous infections, a second attack can produce severe bleeding and even death.

The future appears bleak in regard to global warming. Although the United States is the world's leader in production of greenhouse gases, contributing more than 20 percent of total annual carbon dioxide burden, China, now in second place, is increasing its CO_2 release at a stunning rate (up 27 percent in less than ten years). With understandable determination to become more affluent, China will require a profound increase in energy, almost certainly by use of its abundant supply of coal. That presents a gargantuan problem.

But it is not only the progressive increase in carbon dioxide levels that is of concern. Methane could be an equally important greenhouse gas in the next century. Methane traps heat far more effectively than CO_2. Its sources are much harder to control. They include: swamps, marshes, wetlands, fens, and bogs; coal, oil, and gas extraction; rice paddies; termites; and the intestinal tracts of ruminants. The rule of thumb is for every one billion new people on plant earth, there will be 500 million more cattle; the more cattle, the more methane. Atmospheric concentrations have been increasing sharply for the past 200 years; concentrations have more than doubled since the year 1800, but, for the last ten years, methane concentration has been on a plateau, perhaps because of decreased fossil fuel extraction after the collapse of the Soviet Union. It is likely that levels will again increase in coming decades.

Two consequences of the combination of population increase and global warming are: more poverty and ever-increasing urbanization. Poverty promotes infections, in part, by crowding in unhygienic conditions and, in part, because it leads to malnutrition. Billions of people on this planet suffer some degree of under nutrition or malnutrition, 800 million experience major under nutrition and 400 million suffer dire malnutrition. It used to be thought that malnutrition made the individual (the host) more susceptible by interfering with host defenses against infection. Recent studies suggest that under-nutrition in the host can affect invading microbes, actually making them more venomous by genetic changes in the microbes themselves.

Overpopulation leads to more extensive urbanization. At the start of the 20th century, 15% of the world's population lived in cities. Currently, that has increased to almost 50%; and by the year 2030, an estimated 65% of the approximately 8 billion people on planet Earth will live in cities. Most of these urban centers, particularly in so-called developing countries, will have extensive slums where people are crowded together in unhygienic circumstances, a situation in which mosquito and fly vectors and rodents will thrive, producing the setting for both point source epidemics and rapid person-to-person spread of infectious agents.

Not only are population growth and global climate change in themselves critical issues, but also it is vital to attend to them now, before they get out of hand, because once the population size has become excessive, or the earth has warmed significantly, there is no obvious remedial action. There are many who now believe any problem is amenable to a technologic fix, but, when we have a world population that is too large, any "technologic" solution would take decades or even centuries to succeed, plenty of time for multiple severe emerging infection epidemics, as well as the occurrence of other population size-related catastrophic events. Conceivably, technologic fixes could help reduce carbon dioxide levels in the atmosphere, but, at present, we have no such technologies and reversing global warming would take many decades, if it could be reversed at all.

Given that the two most important societal variables determining the frequency and severity of emerging infection epidemics are population growth and global warming, the actions of the United States Administration and the Congress are bizarre. Population control through family planning has been undercut by reducing funds and by savaging any program that even discusses abortion as one aspect of family planning. We ought to be encouraging every effective family planning program and we should increase our funding of family planning by at least several fold.

The indifference to global warming is equally distressing. The shameful list includes: denial of the scientific evidence of global warming, rejection of the carbon dioxide-controlling Kyoto accord, refusing to enact conservation measures, puny funding for alternative fuels, refusal to commit to renewable energy sources, and an unwillingness to think seriously about the consequences of our indifference. Rejection of Kyoto virtually constitutes criminally negligent behavior.

We cannot prevent all emerging infections epidemics, but we can prevent a large percentage of them and we can mitigate the severity of those that do occur by using a systems approach. With the simpler linear approach, all we can do is react to such epidemics as best we can as they occur and that is hardly satisfactory—it leaves the medical profession in the undesirable position of reacting to epidemics that potentially could have been avoided by effectively attending to major societal determinants.

Illicit Drug Use: For the last fifty years, illicit use of mind-altering drugs has plagued all parts of American society. It spread progressively from 1950 to the mid-1970s. Since then, little has changed, despite massive efforts and expenditure of huge amounts of money. New fads have appeared and faded, use of specific drugs has increased somewhat or decreased somewhat, but overall the chronic use of drugs such as heroin and cocaine is largely unchanged—a societal problem that refuses to go away. There are an estimated 500,000 to one million or more persons dependent on heroin or cocaine in the United States, and millions of heavy users of marijuana and other drugs. The reductionist linear approach by politicians, law enforcement, and the public is to treat or jail individual users and to reduce supply. That approach has not succeeded in the past and never will in the future.

Reducing supply will not succeed so long as there is continuing demand for the drugs by young people and so long as they are willing to pay money for those drugs, thus creating huge profits. If the billion dollar campaign to wipe out the cocaine supply from Colombia were to succeed (it won't), another source of supply would crop up. The same is true of heroin. Cut off one supply route, for example, in Mexico, and another will develop through the Caribbean immediately. And then there are clandestine laboratories manufacturing drugs like ecstasy or methamphetamine. Reducing supply is still worthwhile—we can win individual battles, but we cannot win the war so long as demand is strong.

Then, of course, there are unexpected events that boost production. In Afghanistan, the Taliban reduced opium production by about 80 percent. After they were removed from power, subsistence farmers in rural Afghanistan, impoverished even more than usual by constant war and an implacable drought, found they needed to cultivate opium to survive, and within one year Afghanistan opium production increased dramatically.

We continue to throw non-violent users and small-time drug sellers into prison for extended periods. That is stupid, cruel, and unproductive. They account for more than twenty percent of our jail and prison population, and that is a major reason our jail and prison population now exceeds two million people—at a cost of $20,000 or more per person per year. Building more prisons is not the answer to our drug problem, either.

New York State is among the worst. I was the president of Governor Nelson Rockefeller's Drug Abuse Control Commission and supposedly his top advisor on drugs. He spent $500,000,000 on rehabilitation efforts. When that failed, in frustration and desperation, without adequate consultation, he enacted the draconian, lock-them-up laws that are still in place in New York State. Nelson Rockefeller was an intelligent, compassionate pragmatist. Had he remained governor he would have rescinded those cruel laws decades ago. The prolonged incarceration of non-violent users and small-time sellers (supporting their own habits) is a disgrace that tarnishes any claims of accomplishments by governors and legislators in New York State over the last three decades.

Incarceration is not an intelligent approach to the drug problem—except for major sellers and suppliers and violent drug offenders who should be given long prison sentences. Treatment is the current rage, but it too is largely a mirage. The best that drug free rehabilitation programs for motivated heroin abusers can achieve is about a 35 percent one-year post-treatment abstinence rate; but most heroin users are not motivated to enter drug rehabilitation. The situation is similar with cocaine. Residential programs suffer about a 50 percent dropout rate in the first three months. For those remaining in treatment more than three months, drug use a year after treatment completion drops dramatically, as does criminal behavior; but less than one-third are employed full time, and a significant percentage return to treatment programs. So, treatment may succeed for one-third or fewer of the heroin and cocaine users who are motivated to stop use. There is no reason to believe that compelling "treatment" will succeed for arrested users who are not motivated to undergo treatment and rehabilitation.

We need good treatment and rehabilitation programs, and we desperately need post-treatment support by social workers, counselors, etc. Good programs deserve public and financial support. But treatment is not the answer to our drug problem; it can help, but it is not the answer.

As a consequence of a simplistic linear approach to drug abuse, and in frustration with our inability to mitigate the problem over the last four decades, we have turned to an additional counterproductive policy: coercive drug testing policy for students engaged in athletics and other extracurricular activities. For those urging mandatory urine testing for junior and senior high school athletes, the premise was simple. Do unannounced mandatory urine analysis of athletes for use of marihuana, cocaine, heroin, etc. in the middle schools and the high schools and it will go a long way to controlling substance abuse. About one of every five middle and high schools surveyed have initiated drug testing for athletes and, in some schools, for students involved in other extracurricular activities. Athletes were singled out with rationales that ranged from safety to being good role models with the notion that, if athletes reduced their drug use, the rest of the school body would follow. That notion was used to justify coercive invasion of students' privacy.

There were real consequences for positive findings, including forced counseling and dismissal from the team. Refusal to participate resulted in the student being prevented from participating in athletic activities. The mandatory testing program for student athletes, requiring students to submit to urine tests in order to be allowed to play, was, of course, challenged in court. The case eventually reached the Supreme Court. The Court, in 1995, handed down an extraordinary decision. I have called it The Communal Shower decision. Writing for the majority, Justice Anthony Scalia argued that student athletes took showers together, and taking showers together and or getting dressed for sports in the locker room was proof positive that "school sports are not for the bashful." Because students who participate in sports are allegedly not "bashful" and shower together, they have, according to Scalia, reduced expectations of privacy and it was, therefore, all right to demand they provide urine samples under the watchful eyes of "discrete micturition observers." Taking communal showers according to six members of our Supreme Court was enough to say that these athletes did not deserve the privacy protection of the Fourth Amendment to our Constitution! In 2002, an opinion written by Justice Clarence Thomas reaffirmed this strange reasoning and expanded it to include others engaged in extracurricular activities. According to that bizarre rationale, anyone who is an athletic club member or goes to a camp or does anything else where showers are shared can be hauled off into a booth where a "trained observer" will watch the person urinate so the specimen can be tested for a variety of drugs.

Picking on athletes and others participating in extracurricular activities focuses on the wrong groups. It is the non-participants who are, in actuality, more likely to have uncommitted time to engage in regular illicit drug use. In the absence of probable cause, it is an unethical invasion of privacy. It was instituted without proper studies on the severity of the drug problem in many of the schools adopting it. It can ruin lives because of false positives and the consequences of overreacting to transient experimentation.

Aside from the ethical issue of selecting only students in sports or other extracurricular activities (the ones less likely to use illicit drugs extensively), the obvious question is whether coercive testing does any good. It certainly does nothing but harm for those students who are misidentified by false positive tests. A recent controlled study confirms that drug use is much less frequent among student athletes. Another study, a national sample conducted by the best student drug survey group in the country, found that mandatory urine testing does not reduce student drug use.

The question now is how many schools that have urine testing programs will abandon them on the grounds there is no evidence they do anything other than invade a student's privacy? How many schools will continue testing programs already in existence or will ignore the evidence and start new programs? Will schools about to do testing first require evidence that there is a problem (by doing proper anonymous surveys) and also initiate post-testing evaluation surveys that, considering the frequent fluctuations in the drug scene, must include proper comparison schools in which no drug testing was carried out? My own bet is that most schools with drug testing programs will continue them and more schools will start programs (without surveys) regardless of the evidence. I hope I am wrong. Testing student athletes or those involved in extracurricular activities was and is a bad idea. If testing is to be done, it should be done only on a limited basis and only if there is clear documentation that there is a real problem. Above all, decisions should be based on evidence. And, there is no justification for picking only on athletes or students engaged in other extracurricular activities.

The Fourth Amendment to the Constitution protects privacy only to a very limited extent. That modest degree of protection should be treated with respect, not undercut by strange and bizarre rationalizations for invasion of privacy. We should all remember that rights taken away are not easily restored. When the rights of one group are indiscriminately abrogated, it becomes easier to invade the privacy rights of other groups and eventually there is no privacy for anyone.

Is there a potentially more effective approach? I believe there is. It is inherent in the systems approach. A systems approach is more complex, but offers a greater potential for finding specific interventions that might make a real difference.

Why do young people use illicit mind-altering drugs? There are many reasons. Probably the top three are: curiosity, pleasure, and peer group pressure. It is hardly surprising that curiosity heads the list. A biblical phrase goes "a man should live if only to satisfy his curiosity." Equally unsurprising is pleasure seeking; we are, after all, a hedonistic society focused on both pleasure and instant gratification. Peer groups have an extraordinary influence, for good or bad, on the fragile egos of adolescents seeking acceptance.

The best way to prevent commitment to drugs is to create positive peer pressure by having young people involved in activities that make them feel good about themselves and, at the same time, avoid boredom. Boredom is an invitation to involvement in the drug scene. As Shakespeare noted in Anthony and Cleopatra, "10,000 ills more than the harms I know my idleness doth hatch." The highest juvenile crime period is between the end of school and dinner time—a period in which boredom and peer group pressure dominate.

The proposed remedy is a wide variety of extracurricular activities that should be an intrinsic part of the program of every junior high school and high school, and should be mandatory unless there is a valid excuse. All sorts of activities should be encouraged so that each young person can find something that he or she finds interesting and self-fulfilling. If that is done, it will not prevent experimentation with drugs such as marihuana, but it will markedly reduce serious involvement in the drug scene and it will create constructive peer groups.

We have known this for forty years. I emphasized it in books and articles I wrote in the late 1960s and early 1970s. Despite that knowledge, what have we done as a society in the last three decades? Counterproductively, we have progressively reduced funding for extracurricular activities in our schools, a move that is catastrophic in regard to the drug scene and promotes the influence of unconstructive peer groups. And, the situation is getting worse as local governments face increasing financial pressures and deficits.

Everybody shares the blame—politicians, school boards, members of communities who regularly vote down school budgets, and school administrators who have not formulated adequate plans and have not been effective advocates for extracurricular programs. All these individuals and groups decry the drug scene, but then take actions that promote it. Parents, too, have a responsibility to find interesting, constructive activities that occupy their children.

The systems approach I have illustrated with emerging infections and drug abuse can be used to good advantage for a wide array of problems from terrorism to the potential for extraordinary longevity. Implementing this critical change in our educational system is not difficult. Once students understand and accept the tenets of systems thinking, it gives them the flexibility to adjust to the specific problems at hand, recognizing that some can be approached in a simpler linear fashion whereas others require a broader systems focus. The proposed changes in our education system will not cost a lot of money but will require a change in the way most educators think. Students should not be allowed to graduate from high schools and colleges unless they can demonstrate their competence to take specific problems and put them into a systems context. I submit that no one can be called "educated" in the absence of that capacity.

The future of our society, indeed whether that society has a future, may well depend on how we teach our students, who will become the country's leaders, how to think about the major problems facing their society, and this means that we will almost certainly have to modify our educational system in accord with the three interconnected recommendations I have outlined.

Aging

Profound demographic changes are taking place around the planet that will result in huge numbers of old and very old people. At present, there are 600 million people living on the planet who are over age sixty-five; by the year 2030 that number will increase to 1.3 billion. More than 20 percent of the European—North American population will be over age sixty-five, and more than 5 percent over age eighty. For Asia and Latin America, the figures will be 10 percent over age sixty-five, and 2 percent over age eighty. Africa will have the smallest percentage of older persons—about 5 percent over age sixty-five and 1 percent over eighty. In the United States, by the year 2050 there will be 80 million people, one-fifth of the total population, over age 65, and an incredible 16 to 20 million over age 85.

Faced with this demographic onslaught of older people, the scientific community, despite the best of intentions, is inadvertently going to make the problem worse by creating even larger numbers of old and very old people.

Health professionals and scientists focused on prolonging human life can be divided into two groups: The first group of professionals intends to achieve its goals by controlling major diseases (such as cancer and coronary heart disease) or by reducing some of the deterioration accompanying the ageing process that can promote certain diseases (for example, by using nutritional supplements to slow or reverse the decline in our immune systems that characterizes the aging process).

If the goals of preventing or successfully treating disease are achieved, we might anticipate that average life expectancy at birth would increase to between ninety and one-hundred years, roughly a two decade increase for the "developed" world (average life span currently 76 years) and a three decade increase for the "less developed" world (average life span currently sixty-six years).

The other group of scientists, energized by extraordinary scientific discoveries being reported with ever-increasing frequency, are determined to literally modify the aging process itself and change the boundaries of aging, thus allowing life expectancy at birth to increase in coming decades or centuries to 110 to 120 or more years. The idea, in part, is to decipher the mechanisms underlying aging and then find pharmacologic agents that mimic those mechanisms that promote longevity and interfere with mechanisms that result in reduced longevity. In experimental models, there are multiple promising approaches to extraordinary longevity, including the following:

Reducing caloric intake without producing malnutrition: This extends life spans in many species, including rats and mice. Long-term studies on monkeys suggest that similar life extension will also be found in primates. Now, the race is on to find substances that mimic caloric restriction.

Stimulating certain genes: Genes when stimulated, can start a cascade of events that increases life spans. The most promising substance discovered thus far is resveratrol, found in red wines. Resveratrol has extended life spans in fruit flies and mice. Studies on other genes and the peptides they produce are equally hopeful.

Interfering with genes (so-called gene knockout studies) that promote aging: This, on the basis of yeast and mouse studies, looks quite promising.

Stem cells: Then there is the potential of stem cells to replace worn out tissues, including heart muscle and brain. Others are investigating telomerase-like agents that can keep the telomeres at the end of chromosomes long. Because cell aging is associated with progressive shortening of the telomeres, keeping them long could theoretically keep these cells viable and young indefinitely.

Nanotechnology: For the perhaps not-too-distance future, there is the promise of nanotechnology and the possibility that nanorobots in our blood streams could maintain our homeostasis, correcting mutations, preventing buildup of arteriosclerotic plaques in blood vessels, in essence, keeping us young.

Scientific advances in this area are stunning and progress in both areas (maximizing physiologic life span and changing the boundaries of aging) are so spectacular that the possibility for human application of these animal, insect, and test tube studies in the near future by responsible scientists and physicians is very real.

At present, despite talk about anti-aging agents or cocktails, there is no substance that has been shown in humans to extend life span by even a single day. But, given the astounding progress, it is inevitable that successful experimental models will be tried in humans. My own view is that it is only a matter of time before we are able to create very old people, allowing average life expectancy at birth to increase to 100, 110, or 120 years. To me, it is not a question of whether we will be able to do it, but when.

It could be that maximizing physiologic life spans or changing the boundaries of aging will be a huge boon to humankind with most people living longer, healthier, and happier lives, but a systems approach to the societal consequences raises the following questions and concerns that relate to very old people, to the local or national society, and to the global society.

1. The world population is now more than six billion people. If scientific endeavors are successful, at the dawn of the next century there could be two or three people on this planet for every one we have now, and more than one-third the population could be over sixty years of age. Each decade extension of life expectancy will add at least 1.3 billion people to the eventual population of planet Earth. If average life expectancy around the world can be increased by four decades from the current 66 years to 106 years, that would add 5 billion people resulting in a world population at stability of 15 billion instead of the currently projected 10 billion persons. That raises two derivative questions:

   • At what point is the world population so large that it exceeds the carrying capacity of the planet, thus sowing the seeds for our own destruction?
   • At what point does the crush of human numbers make life miserable for the vast majority of humans and impossible for many other species?

2. In the United States, at present, 13% of the population (the 37 million people over age 65) consumes about 33% of health care dollars. What happens when 30 percent are over age 65?

Would they consume 75 % of health care dollars? That would be unacceptable; indeed, it would be unthinkable.

3. Will a large percentage of old and very old people outlive their financial resources and spend decades in poverty? The percentage of older persons considered to be living in poverty or near poverty in the United States doubles between ages 65 and 85. A large percentage of older people depend, in substantial part or virtually completely, on Social Security. By 2050, the ratio of active workers to retirees is expected to fall from the present 3:1 to 2:1. Unless immigration is markedly increased, the ratio will continue to fall and even-tually the Social Security system will become non-viable.

4. Will older people be expected to remain in the work force until age seventy, or eighty, or one-hundred? The official age of retirement will soon increase from 65 to 67 years. Politi-cians and economists debate, often acrimoniously, about potential further increases to ages 68, 69, or 70. If average expected life span increases to 100 to 120 years, there will have to be a re-thinking of the whole concept of retirement. Many people out of financial necessity may have to work far beyond the usual retirement age. Many others, recognizing their likely long period of survival after age 65 or 70, may wish to work out of choice, unwilling or ill-suited to have three to five decades of additional life expectancy without employment activity. This, in turn, will potentially create a severe inter-generational adversarial situation as young, mid-dle aged, old, and very old people compete for a limited number of jobs, a problem that may be compounded by technologic advances that reduce the need for human employees.

5. Will extended longevity be accompanied by overall health or will those extended years be compromised by decrements such as profoundly reduced vigor, impaired mental function, dysfunctional muscles and joints? Will those anti-aging pills succeed in keeping only parts of us young? It is implausible that an anti-aging pill or injection will, in some miraculous fashion, be a panacea, obviating all or even most of the irri-tating and sometimes debilitating decrements that accom-pany chronologic aging. Certainly it will not stop the herniated discs or the postoperative infections following back surgery, knee, and hip surgery, etc. If this human

regeneration is only partial, the gift of extra years could be disastrous. The optimists would have us believe these centenarians-plus will retain youthful mental and physical vigor and virility, fully engaged in their society. That may be true for some but what if for a large percentage of the very old, the youthful vigor promised to them is a mirage and instead, with inadequate financial resources they are no longer able to live with their children, grandchildren, or great grandchildren, they are warehoused into facilities for people of similar age, frail of body, mind, or spirit, bored, focused almost monolithically on body function and waiting with increasing impatience for the finality of death? Obviously, quality of life as longevity is extended is a critical issue.

I have painted a potentially grim picture of future consequences of anti-aging endeavors. There is no intention to denigrate the scientific efforts or achievements. The scientific investigations of the mechanisms of aging and the studies on changing life spans in experimental models by a variety of techniques are marvelous. They should be supported and nurtured by additional funding. But, there has been none of the necessary societal debate—not a good idea.

We need biologic scientists, ethicists, philosophers, demographers, theologians, historians, economists, politicians, social scientists, psychologists, among others, to become much more interested in the potential consequences of our astounding and accelerating scientific achievements in the area of aging. We need to figure out how to keep older people, if they wish, in the job market and we have to figure out how to keep them involved in society. Social Security will likely have to be replaced. It may be necessary to place restrictions on drugs or technologies that could result in extraordinary longevity extension.

Significant increase in average life spans (to 90 or 95 years) by better disease prevention and treatment is virtually guaranteed, and that is good. Extraordinary longevity (to 100 to 120 years) is another story. It is no longer science fiction. We must prepare or we will be dragged willy-nilly to our demographic destiny, and we will be likely to encounter some very unpleasant circumstances when we get there.

Health Care

The final issue I shall discuss relates to what can be done about our extraordinarily expensive health care system.

It seems inevitable that the United States will eventually have to turn to a single payer system, to some form of national health insurance. The current system, now costing $1.8 trillion annually, more than $5,000 per person, is unwieldy and inefficient; and it will get worse as costs increase due to an aging population and the development of ever more sophisticated (and expensive) technologies and pharmacologic agents. The annual costs will approach $3 trillion by 2012, and that will almost certainly force change to a system that is far more efficient than the one we have now—and that means some sort of national health insurance. The critical and unanswered question is what percentage of gross national product is the American public willing to devote to health care? If it is, for example, 20 percent of gross national product, instead of the current 14 percent, we will have to make choices. If a lot more is spent on health, less will be available to spend elsewhere (e.g., on the military).

No matter what happens with the organization of medical care, we will have to become more efficient and approach both disease prevention and treatment more economically based on evidence. Probably one-half the costly examinations, tests, and procedures currently carried out are unnecessary. That includes the vast majority of annual physical examinations and automated laboratory tests. The routine annual physical examination has not been shown to be beneficial?—but, it makes substantial amounts of money for health care professionals and so it is still popular, even though ineffective.

If we did only the examinations, procedures, and tests that are really needed and beneficial, we could save tens of billions of dollars each year. In regard to health promotion and disease prevention, the Health Wellness Promotion Act developed in New Jersey has a limit on required expenditures to carry out the tests and actions. It is a reasonable limit that increases annually in accord with the Consumer Price Index. That ceiling is essential for health promotion and disease prevention; we have to get the job done and yet limit the expenditures. The cap on required expenditures establishes the principle that we will pay for documented health promotion–disease prevention. If an individual wishes additional, but inadequately documented, tests or procedures, that is all right, but it must be paid for by supplemental insurance or out of pocket, or an insurer or managed care organization may offer the test or procedure for public relations (or other) reasons. The cap also means that, in future years when we have more documented disease prevention tests and procedures than can be fitted under the cap, the individual and health care provider will have to figure out what is best for that individual at that particular time given a limit on the amount that can be spent in that year on health promotion–disease prevention. We have to make choices and these choices should be based on evidence. Under the Health Wellness Promotion Act at present, for example, screening for prostate cancer is not included, and it will not be until there is clear evidence that finding cancers by the blood test PSA (prostate specific antigen) actually saves lives or significantly prolongs good quality life.

Health promotion–disease prevention will not succeed fully unless it can effectively intervene in three intertwined American epidemics—overweight and obesity, physical inactivity, and diabetes. In my judgment, a very good start would be at annual comprehensive prevention examinations. At that examination, weight, dietary intake, and physical activity can be determined, counseling performed, and, where appropriate, healthy behavior change initiated.

I feel reasonably optimistic about health care. I believe the increasing costs will force us to adopt a better health care system and insist on evidence-based health care, more efficient treatment, and a greater focus on health promotion–disease prevention. I wish I felt as optimistic about the global society. I am a Futurist and futurists draw up alternative scenarios for future years or decades (or centuries). Planning for the future, by definition, requires some optimism. After all if you spend time planning for the future, you must have a modicum of faith that there will be a future. Our technologic cornucopia could give us a much better future, but technologic advances have the capacity to both benefit and harm mankind (the airplane, for example); so, I am not a devotee of the notion that technologic advances will solve all problems and not be used for massively destructive purposes. What is needed is a combination of an educated public, thinking like futurists, using a systems approach for complex issues, and tackling societal problems, such as population excess and global warming, before there is a crisis. We will also have to reduce the disparity between the haves and the have-nots on this planet, and we must embrace the concept of sustainability, defined as one genration not depleting natural resources or damaging the planet to the detriment of succeeding generations. All that, in turn, requires much better local, national, and global leadership than we have now. We simply cannot afford politicians and leaders with rigid ideologies or those interested primarily in themselves and their personal advancement with virtually a monolithic focus on the next election or staying in power. If the education system, here and in other countries, instills the systems thinking approach to problems, then in a generation or so we are likely to have politicians and leaders who think well enough to enable our American society and the global society to not only survive, but also to thrive.

Winston Churchill said: "What is the use of living if it be not to make this muddled world a better place to live in after we are gone?"

That takes foresight, planning, and leadership. Will we follow that Churchillian precept? I do not know, but for the sake of my children, my grandchildren, and their children—and all the rest of the children and grandchildren on this beleaguered planet, I hope we will.

Dr. Louria trained in internal medicine at the New York Hospital. He then began an academic career in infectious diseases, first at the National Institutes of Health and then at Cornell's Infectious Disease Unit at Bellevue Hospital. Subsequent interest in drug abuse led to his appointment as head of Governor Nelson Rockefeller's drug abuse program. Dr. Louria subsequently became Professor & Chairman of the Department of Preventive Medicine and Community Health, New Jersey Medical School. He remains a full time faculty member, focusing his attention on major public health and education policy issues.

The Cultural, Situational, and Social Contexts of Health and Disease

P. Herbert Leiderman

I dedicate this essay to my youngest daughter Andrea N. Leiderman, B.A., M.P.P. who died at age 46 on September 11, 2005. She was indefatigable in her political and professional career in bringing health and educational services to the underserved members of our community, best exemplifying what a "caring and responsible" citizen can accomplish even in her shortenedlife span.

> *"Life is not what one lived, but what one remembers, and how one remembers it in order to recount it."*
>
> —Gabriel García Márquez

Personal History

I was born on January 30, 1924, in Chicago, Illinois, to parents born in England who had come to the United States as infants. Their parents (my grandparents) migrated to the United States from the Ukraine, then part of Czarist Russia, in the 1890s, escaping from the pogroms against Jews then common in that region. My paternal grandparents, who had an urban background, migrated directly to Chicago, where my grandfather continued his trade as a cigar maker. My maternal grandparents, residents of a "*shtetl*" village, migrated to rural western Michigan, where they settled on the government land provided to railroads as an incentive to promote the building of the railways. The land was poor for agriculture. My grandfather was fortunate in that he could use his other skills as a machinist, learned while he was a recruit in the Russian army in Warsaw in the 1880s. He was a railroad machinist until 1935, an ardent member of the union with an abiding hatred for Russians, whether "red" or "white."

My father trained in the law but never practiced his profession, leaving it in favor of his primary love of sports, much to his parents' chagrin. He became a recreation director for the Chicago Public Parks, assigned to the Maxwell Street/Hull House district, in an immigrant ghetto. He worked from 1 to 10 P.M. five days a week and all day on Saturday. I rarely saw him except on Saturdays, when I would spend part or all of the day at the park with him. I became acquainted with ethnic diversity, urban poverty, and ethnic conflict during these Saturday visits.

My mother's family moved to Chicago in 1917 after my mother's graduation from high school in Muskegon, Michigan. My mother trained as a librarian at the Library School of the Chicago Public Library and met my father at a public park where both were employed. My mother was a member of the "radical" John Reed Club and an active feminist who marched in the feminist parades of 1919/1920 in Chicago. She was widely read, a social and politically engaged woman, definitely not concerned with household chores. However, she was concerned about her children's education, visited the local primary school often, made certain my sister and I read books, took us to museums and regularly to the children's theater at the famed Goodman in Chicago.

I count three transforming experiences in my early life: first the economic Depression of 1929–1937; second my parents' ownership of a children's summer camp from 1936 to 1956, and third was World War II, 1941–45, all of which profoundly shaped my beliefs, values, attitudes, and perhaps even behavior.

The first of these was growing up in ethnic Chicago during the Depression, and because of my father's work and my mother's political interests, I became well acquainted with urban poverty and very aware of social class and ethnic differences. When visiting my father on Saturdays, I observed men and women on street corners who appeared to own nothing more than the torn and ragged clothes covering their bodies. Destitute children, chiefly black with an admixture of Mexicans and whites, were openly begging on the streets.

My view of American poverty continued during my father's two weeks of vacation every summer. Our family spent part of every August traveling by car to various parts of the Midwest; on one occasion we went west to Pike's Peak and on another east to Washington, DC. Whether or not my parents intended it, my experience of poverty was reinforced by visits to the striking coal miners of Harlan County, Kentucky, the poverty-stricken folk of the Missouri Ozarks, the poor "colored" folk living in the urban slums behind the Capitol in Washington, DC., dustbowl farmers of the Midwest, and the destitute Ojibway Indians of Wisconsin and Sioux Indians of South Dakota. Although I do not believe this "tour of poverty" was a deliberate effort by my parents to educate my sister and me about America, it did make me aware amidst "fun" travel that there were people less fortunate than we, and that we should try to help them as much as possible. Charity and concern for the less fortunate were guiding principles in my upbringing.

A second transforming experience, which influenced my career choice in teaching and subsequent clinical interest in medicine, was participation in a family-operated children's summer camp. My parents started a private camp in order to supplement my father's civil service income. From 1936 to 1956 my mother fulfilled her personal ambitions by directing the camp, located in rural south-central Michigan. Except for the war years of 1942–1945, all of my free time on weekends and all summers from 1936 to 1953 were involved with the camp. This experience set the stage for my later professional life, kindling my interest in families and children; I learned to take care of people in trouble, develop a pragmatic outlook, and solve problems under any and all conditions.

The third and perhaps the most transforming experience related to my subsequent career was my university education and military experience during WWII. My first choice for higher education beyond high school was the University of Chicago, whose reputation as judged by my peers was in the first rank. I was accepted in 1941 but could not attend for financial reasons. My next option was the University of Michigan, where I applied and was accepted, majoring in physics and mathematics.

WW II for the United States began in December 1941, my freshman year. I made the decision in November 1942 to join the Army Air Corps Reserve with the intention of pilot training, encouraged by the Army's promise that I could complete my second year at Michigan before going into service. Shortly thereafter I transferred into a special seven-month pre-meteorology program at the University of New Mexico, and upon completion of the course was transferred to the meteorology program at the

California Institute of Technology. I graduated as a second lieu-tenant on June 5, 1944. I was assigned to the North Atlantic Area, where I spent the next two years forecasting weather for the North Atlantic region, northern New England, Canada, Green-land, Iceland, Scotland, and England.

I spent most of my military career (two winters and two sum-mers) in the sub-arctic climate at Goose Bay, Labrador, and a few months in western Newfoundland before discharge in July 1946. At ages 20 to 22, I, along with my colleagues, six officers and twenty-five enlisted men, were responsible for the success of flights, chiefly bombers, going off to Scotland and England to prepare for eventual missions over Europe. As meteorologists we performed the technical work of forecasting weather under highly stressful conditions with inadequate data, using rudimen-tary scientific principles, predicting the "future" and being eval-uated every day for our success or failure. I learned to take responsibility for decision-making at an early stage of my adult-hood. It turned out to be excellent preparation for a career in medicine, though I did not fully appreciate this aspect of my training until I entered internship and residency programs after medical school.

I was discharged from service in July 1946; I had spent an extra year in service after being declared "essential" by the Army Air Corps. With the famed GI Bill in hand, I entered the univer-sity of my first choice: the University of Chicago. I decided not to continue in the physical sciences. I felt the issues for our country and the world could more likely be dealt with by knowl-edge of the social and the behavioral sciences rather than my work in physics. The Holocaust was prominent in my thoughts, reinforced by military-sponsored travel to England, France, Ger-many, Czechoslovakia, and Italy after the war and viewing the incredible damage wrought by the bombers we had sent on to England. I was brought face to face with man's inhumanity to man. I felt that understanding human behavior would give me a better chance to make a difference in doing something about this tragedy.

At this juncture biosocial imperatives came to the fore. I met through mutual friends a recent graduate of the University of Illi-nois in sociology who had grown up in the Chicago suburbs under social conditions of minority status and social isolation, similar to my own childhood experiences. Gloria Frank and I met, decided we were suited for one another, fell in love, and married in November 1947. Both of us attended graduate school together at the University of Chicago from 1947 to 1949, working on degrees in human development and psychology.

In 1947 James G. Miller, M.D., Ph.D. (Harvard), was appointed chairman of Psychology department at the University of Chicago. He encouraged me to consider a career path combining the M.D. and Ph.D. degrees because of my clinical interests. He suggested I apply to Harvard Medical School, though being a Midwesterner I preferred to remain in Chicago. To my surprise I was accepted by Harvard, leaving me with a choice between Chicago and Harvard. My wife applied to the Ph.D. Program in Child Development at Harvard and was accepted.

With both acceptances in hand, we made the decision to be off to Boston for only four years. We both received our graduate degrees (M.D. and Ph.D.) in June 1953, with our parents and my maternal grandparents in attendance. Ten years later, after residency training in neurology and psychiatry, and additional postdoctoral experience, four children, one dog, and two cats, we left Boston to follow the Horace Greeley injunction, "Go West, young man!" (and woman), this time all the way, stopping in the Midwest only briefly. We have been at Stanford University ever since.

Contextual Research and Clinical Medicine

Both my research interests and my clinical activities have reflected my social/behavioral orientation in medicine—particularly the contexts influenced by cultural, situational, and social class factors. My earliest studies on situational context began while I was a resident in neurology at Boston City Hospital. They stemmed from my clinical experience in treating "Iron Lung Psychosis"; that is, hallucinatory behavior in poliomyelitis patients who were confined in respirators because of thoracic muscular paralysis. It turned out that the social isolation and sensory deprivation of confinement to a respirator was the likely explanation of the phenomenon. When we provided sensory stimulation and social relationships to the patients, the psychosis disappeared.

After moving to the Stanford Medical School's Department of Psychiatry, I began a second study on situational factors influencing human behavior. I became co-principal investigator in a 3-year project studying the effect of delayed mother and infant contact in the newborn period. My colleagues had observed that mothers of premature infants often had difficulty in mothering when they were reunited with their infants after the babies were discharged from the premature nursery. The difficulty was attributed in part to the delayed social bonding of a mother with her infant, because the mother and infant were separated while the infant was in the premature newborn nursery. We hypothesized that a critical period might exist for maternal social bonding to an infant, analogous to that seen in some mammalian species, particularly sheep and goats, where early separation decreased subsequent maternal bonding. To test the hypothesis, my colleagues and I manipulated the social environment of the premature nursery at six-month intervals, permitting mothers and premature infants to be in contact in one situation, and maintaining the usual premature nursery separation in the second situation. Neither group of mothers was aware of the other group, as the entire nursery was changed for 6-month intervals over a 2-year period.

The results revealed some effects of delayed separation, mainly less close physical contact by mother with infant after reunion, more anxiety, and heightened concern for the infant. These effects were somewhat attenuated by nine months after reunion. We found no evidence for a critical period in human mother–infant bonding. Prematurity itself had some effect on maternal behavior regardless of separation, mainly tentative and anxious behavior when compared to mothers of full term infants.

These results led to major changes in premature nurseries throughout the United States: All mothers of premature infants now are allowed early contact with their infants if they prefer to do so. There appeared to be no harmful effects for infants (i.e., infection) with their mothers' presence in the nursery, and considerable psychosocial benefits for the mothers.

An example of the influence of familial and economic contexts on infant development is illustrated by my work in Kenya, East Africa. I planned to continue my observations on mothers and infants during a sabbatical year in Kenya in an agricultural community where close physical contact of mother with infant was the reputed norm. My assumption, based on colleagues' reports, was that mothers in agricultural communities had close physical and social contact, hence strong bonding with their infants from birth onward.

My research assistants and I studied seventy mothers and infants over a one-year period, recording economic status and educational level of families directly observing mothers' daily caretaking and other activities, and measuring infants' growth and cognitive and psychosocial development over a nine month period. I set up clinic in the village, providing services to the mothers and infants, staffed by a trained Kikuyu nurse, a trained Kikuyu family physician, and me. The clinic met once a week for routine problems and as well to collect data on infants and observe maternal caretaking. The usual infant mortality in the village was about ten percent. We lost no infants in the one-year period! We believe the high survival rate of infants was not due solely to our "bush medicine" clinical care, but more likely to the mothers' enthusiasm about our shared interest in their infants.

The study results produced several surprises for me. First, the primary social caretakers of infants turned out to be young girls aged five to ten years old, usually an older daughter or mother's younger sister. Mothers provided breast-feeding and overall management, but the principal social stimulation for the infants was provided by the youthful female baby-minders. Mothers were much too busy with subsistence agriculture and hauling water to the household compound to have much social time for their infants. A second surprise was the finding of the effect of socio-economic class, as measured by size of household plot and mother's education. As little as two years of mothers' attendance in primary school, and residence on larger (two to four acres) land plots had a positive relationship to infants' physical and psychosocial development in infants' first year. A third surprise was the absence of a paternal effect. A small number of fathers resided regularly on the family homestead. These families did not differ from those without a father present. All infants did well despite paternal absence. Father's role became important for male children after age seven when they moved into father's house on the homestead. Siblings and peers turned out to be the most potent socializers for infants in this polymatric caretaking system. The contextual factors of polymatric infant caretaking, maternal educational level, and family economic status (unrelated to infant nutritional status, since all but four infants were well nourished) proved to be important in accounting for the infant's physical and psychological development in the first year.

Context and Social Class in the Real World:
The California Youth Authority

> *"There is nothing in man's plight that his vision,*
> *if he cared to cultivate it, cannot alleviate. The challenge*
> *is to see what could be done, and then to have the*
> *heart and the resolution to attempt it."*
>
> —"George Kennan at 100," N.Y. Review of Books,
> April 29, 2004

The contextual influences of social class status are illustrated in my clinical activities at the California Youth Authority (CYA).

My alarm noisily rouses me at 6.00 A.M., an hour earlier than the usual time. Thus begins my once- or twice-monthly trips of ninety miles to the CYA located in the Central Valley at Stockton, California. The journey is familiar, as I have made it for twenty-four years, but it has been more pleasant because of my wife's companionship since her retirement ten years ago. We have the opportunity to talk without outside interruption and she has the time at our local hotel to read without disturbance while I am at work. Travel to the Central Valley provides both of us with the opportunity to see lifestyles very different from those in the Bay Area, broadening our perspective on the diverse ethnic population of working class and middle-class folk in the Central Valley. We have even become sufficiently familiar with locals, including the security staff at the Youth Authority, to discuss liberal politics in this politically conservative area of California.

The California Youth Authority has custody of youths, typically ages 13–18 (though occasionally older), who have been found guilty of serious crimes, such as murder, rape, assault, or burglary, as well as crimes involved with the use of illegal substances, such as marijuana, cocaine, alcohol, and or methamphetamines. These young men have graduated into the state correctional system after having failed individual and group counseling in the local community, placement in supervised group homes, or incarceration in county closed units at Juvenile Hall. The CYA inmates are predominantly urban, African American, and Mexican American in heritage, with a small admixture of rural Anglo-American whites from the Central Valley, Native Americans from the reservations and nearby towns, and Asians (Cambodians, Hmong, Laotians) from the smaller cities of the Central Valley. They uniformly come from lower-class backgrounds. The vast majority of the youngsters have grown up in poverty-stricken homes where attentive care has been minimal. Single-parent (usually mother) families are frequent, and drug abuse by male and female parents is common. School attendance is intermittent, or non-existent, after grade seven. Organized recreational activities are not available in their communities. Family resources are minimal, barely keeping up with survival needs. Ties to community institutions such as religious organizations and memberships in sports or recreation clubs are rare or absent. Primary (family) or secondary (peer) social attachments are rudimentary except for gang memberships, where some socialization occurs—unfortunate because all too often this socialization is antisocial as judged by the usual community standards.

The staff reflects the ethnic diversity of California, with slight overrepresentation of Anglo-Americans in the professional group, though my child psychiatric colleague is of African-American heritage. About one third of staff—professionals, parole officers, youth counselors, and security officers—are female. I consult with the staff about problem cases (youngsters who are not progressing in the program) and evaluate youths when there is disagreement among the staff about their readiness for discharge into the community. My task is to assess a youth in one interview and write a report to the parole board with my opinion, which is to be used along with other sources of information for their decision whether to discharge the youth into the community.

Over my twenty-four years of consultation in one of the better schools in the Youth Authority system, I have been deeply impressed with the professionalism and dedication of the staff as they attempt to rehabilitate these unfortunate youths. With few exceptions they take their jobs seriously, trying to find ways to make up for years of abuse and neglect and to instill a bit of humanity in youngsters who have had little experience of it. Despite two years or more of incarceration, the task seems almost impossible. The youths can be held until age eighteen, then either discharged or moved to a more restrictive institution in the Youth Authority if they are deemed at risk for re-offense.

One might ask what possible gains we make by incarcerating them. There are some. Many of these young men enter the institution reading at the second or third grade levels. Most aspire to read and many will reach the fifth and sixth grade levels within a year, because in the California Youth Authority system school attendance and homework are mandatory. Special education and individual educational programs are available and used for those with special needs. A few of the youths who have longer sentences will enter a full high school program, graduating with a diploma, and many others will earn a General Education certificate. Practically all the young men (both gang- and non-gang-affiliated) learn to live in an agreeable manner in a socially diverse environment, with due consideration for members of other ethnic, racial, and non-home-based peer groups. Transgressions lead to time additions to their sentences, a significant deterrent to antisocial activity. Many of the youths, though not all, will adopt socially appropriate behavior in relating to female staff. However, comfort with gay or pedophilic peers is still problematic. About 10%–15% of the youths need and receive psychological or psychiatric help with counseling and psychotherapy for post-traumatic stress disorder, depression, attention deficit hyperactivity disorder, or addictive disorders.

The program succeeds with many of these youngsters while they are incarcerated. The problem begins with discharge into the community; by estimate about sixty to seventy percent re-offend and are incarcerated in other institutions within the three-year period after release. The problem is lack of preparation for employment, a return to the communities and situations where they developed their anti-social activities, the lack of post-discharge supervision, and most important, lack of a warm and accepting positive social network.

What I have learned? First, I learned anew about the deficiencies of our current political/social/economic system: We offer little help for children and their families in the earliest years to move youngsters onto a healthier trajectory toward a socially responsible, satisfying, and fulfilling adult life. The current American system simply does not provide for the 10%–15% of the community who for various reasons cannot make their own way in the society. Families, the neighborhood, and the community do not provide the help needed to prevent social pathology for this group, whose numbers may even increase as the psychological/cognitive demands of our complex world increase in this era of overwhelming stimulation.

What should be done? Aspects of good social programs exist in many countries, though to my knowledge there is not a full program in any single country. Sweden, Denmark, and France connect social workers or nurses to practically all families with infants and young children under the age of two. There are low-cost nursery schools for all children to age six or seven. Services for high-risk children are available for preschool and school age children. Services beyond the preschool age in general are less available, but are more available than in the United States.

In the United States services for high risk children are not available. We also need programs for normal children after age ten where parenting is problematic because of employment, divorce, or sheer inadequacy of parental skills amidst very unfavorable environments. For this age group through mid- to late adolescence, school-supervised programs and recreational, academic, athletic, and artistic clubs should be a constituent part of our educational programs, but with a separate, competent staff. Such programs might be voluntary for most adolescents, but for high-risk youths they should be strongly encouraged, with an appropriate reward structure for participation.

Goal-directed vocational programs (alongside academic programs) should be encouraged in high school for students who lack motivation and interest in more abstract learning. These programs could use older peer mentors and part-time supervisors who are paid for this work with money or vouchers for further education, while they continue their own programs in college, university, or professional school.

Implementing a program like the one I have sketched will be extremely difficult in the United States, where external regulation and oversight carry a cultural taboo. Our society does not seem to weigh the losses to the community incurred by ignoring the risks facing youths in the lower socioeconomic classes against the benefits to be gained from support of their social infrastructure. It should be obvious that those from the upper social classes must pay proportionally a greater amount of taxes, which along with whatever taxes derive from the lower classes to pay for the social infrastructure. Though the current societal focus frequently avoids monetary support for long-term projects, I remain in the camp of George Kennan, with some optimism for the future because of the presence of a small group of people who accept the challenge to ". . . see what could be done, and then have the heart and resolution to attempt it."

The Interactive Influences of Context and Culture:
An East African Encounter

A transforming experience both intellectually and professionally was our family decision to spend a 1969/70 sabbatical year in Kenya, East Africa, doing research on mother–infant relationships in a Kikuyu village. This research on mother-to-infant bonding and infant-to-mother social attachment relationships grew out of my research on maternal social bonding with premature infants in the premature infant nursery at Stanford Medical Center. Through contacts at Harvard University I was appointed Field Director of the Child Development Research Unit at University of Nairobi, a program of cross-cultural research on children in Kenya and the United States under the overall direction of Professors John and Beatrice Whiting of Harvard. The Whitings had known of my work on mother–infant social bonding at Stanford through my wife, who had been a graduate student in their program at Harvard. Their need for a research director in the field was a good fit with my plans for forthcoming sabbatical year.

My wife and I were enthusiastic about this opportunity; our children were somewhat suspicious about spending a year away from home and their friends. To prepare as much as possible, we had a weekly Saturday luncheon date at home learning Swahili with a Kenyan–Tanzanian couple, graduate students at Stanford. Our four children did just fine, learning enough Swahili to help us in the village and travel in the "bush." The two adults tried hard, finally managing greetings and names of foods.

In June 1969, four children, aged ten to fifteen years, and two adults began one of the great experiences of their lives. We spent ten weeks traveling in Europe and Israel before arriving in Nairobi in late August 1969. We remained in Africa for an entire year. My role was to serve as field director for four research sites in Kenya. The overall research program for the Whiting project was to examine the social development of children aged 6–12 in four villages scattered throughout Kenya and two communities in the United States. Standard protocols for the samples of children in each community had already been completed, including our Kikuyu agricultural village. In addition to the data set, my wife and I could do additional studies on the same population or other children in our village. Apart from our research, we served as mentors, resource persons, and cheerleaders for graduate student research couples in the more remote sites in rural Kenya.

The project headquarters was located in the so-called white highlands forty miles from Nairobi. The village where we worked was about five miles away from our headquarters homestead, located in a "native" reserve approachable by a mud and gravel road, which in the rainy seasons became almost impassable. At the time of Kenyan independence in 1963 the village was a substantial agricultural community of about 2500 people.

We lived in the field headquarters house, an old stone British settler residence of many rooms, heated by fireplaces, simply furnished, with adequate water and sewage facilities. The house was at 7500 feet elevation, extremely pleasant during the dry season, but cold, damp, drizzly, dark and miserable during the rainy season. Three servants—a cook, an inside man, and an outside man, none of whom could be dismissed because of local custom—came with the house. They lived in their own very simple quarters away from the main house, while their wives and children remained in their home villages. We soon learned how essential their services were, especially when they were absent on a visit to their home villages. We could not have survived without their help.

In addition to our family, four young Kikuyu women aged eighteen to twenty from other parts of Central Kenya lived with us for the year. They were recent graduates of the premier Kenyan high school for native young women and were to serve as our research assistants in the village before going on to the University of Nairobi. For eleven months our breakfast and dinner table comprised ten people: the four young women, three from villages and one from Nairobi, plus our four children, Gloria, and me. Despite differences in backgrounds, generations, and culture, we lived and socialized together with surprising good humor and tolerance, including a ten-day safari to the Masaai Mara, Serengeti, Ngorongoro, and Amboseli game parks in Kenya and Tanzania.

The main effect of this experience was on our family, and as we later learned, on our research assistants. Our family gained perspective on a world very different from our own, which quite likely led to a shift in our career orientation after our return. I dropped a somewhat narrow, ideologically oriented, psychoanalytically derived formulation of human development and turned toward a cultural and social orientation with a clinical interest to working with families and their children. My wife shifted from work in a classical child-developmental mode to a more clinical orientation, becoming for the next nineteen years director of the Palo Alto Peninsula Children's Center devoted to children and adolescents at high risk and with special education needs. Of our four children, three became involved with various aspects of the medical and health care system.

Two of our children, a son and daughter, became physicians, both with a strong public health orientation. Our youngest daughter became head of the Community Affairs Program for Kaiser Permanente in Santa Clara and San Mateo counties. Our other daughter turned toward a creative writing career in rural California. Two of her published stories were about Kenya.

Perhaps more unexpected (and extremely exciting for us) were the career paths of our four female research assistants, all of whom went on to university, and two of whom went on to graduate school and received advanced degrees. As of last year their positions were:

1. Professor of Public Health, University of Nairobi; B.A. University of Nairobi, Kenya, Ph.D. Harvard University.
2. Associate Director African Section, Women's Affairs, World Bank, Washington, D.C.; B.A. University of Nairobi, Kenya
3. Professor of Biology, University of Makerere, Kampala; Ph.D. Uganda
4. Public Affairs Officer, Ministry of Foreign Affairs, Nairobi, Kenya; B.A. Kenya

How or why these young women chose their careers I can only surmise. Two of them with whom we have been in contact attribute their choices in part to our experiences together. I have no doubt this was partially true, judging from the effects of the experience on my family. These young women were intelligent, hard working, ambitious, and conscientious about their research duties. We spent many evenings together around the fireplace discussing almost everything a family does and thinks about, as well as our research work. Our two older daughters, aged thirteen and fifteen, lived in the same portion of the house with these women, and they developed an independent close relationship with our assistants. Whatever happened in the larger household, and however it happened in these relationships, the result was one of the most gratifying aspects of our African experience.

I returned to our Kikuyu village in 1972, and began a second project with colleagues in Western Kenya among the Gusii people in 1974 and 1976. I used these opportunities to travel extensively in Francophone and Anglophone Central and West Africa, especially visiting psychiatric facilities with the goal of finding possible candidates suitable for advanced fellowships in the United States. I learned a great deal in Africa about the power of traditional healing, both alone and combined with Western approaches to psychiatric care. I was impressed with the power of family and community and with cultural support in helping the healing process. Though my quest for candidates for fellowships was unsuccessful—it was too early in the process of professional development to bring candidates to the United States—I came away with the thought that there was much to be gained for our mental health system from the African system of family and community caretaking of the mentally ill.

As a byproduct of my extensive travels, I became acquainted with the political and economic effects of the transition from colonialism to independence in several countries, and very well acquainted with the deficiencies of quasi-democratic political forms engrafted onto traditional communities. I concluded that the few elite, educated Africans who captured economic and political power after independence were not prepared to share power or show concern for the people in the villages. The typical pattern was control of the national Capital and the financial resources of the country by a "Big Man" with his tribesmen, exploiting and terrorizing the majority of the population, who only wanted to survive, take care of and educate their children, and eventually to flourish in conditions of security.

I was particularly impressed with the positive role of women in fostering social and economic development, in sharp contrast to the male members of the community. I came to the conclusion that positive social change was dependent on women's education and support for their well-being. Men seemed concerned with the "immediate"; women more concerned with the "present and future." Further, the World Bank made the grand mistake of focusing on the elites, mainly men like themselves, as partners in this management. The "top-down" approach simply did not work. But even a newer focus on "bottom-up" instead of "top-down" in international development, will take at least two generations for substantial economic, political, and social development to occur in Africa, and then only if women are permitted and encouraged to be participants in the process.

Context and Education of Doctors

At this point I would like to elaborate on the concept of context, because it is critical to understanding my approach to medicine. By adding the concept of context to clinical medicine I want to emphasize that our understanding of pathological processes cannot rely on biological concepts alone. Emphasizing biological explanations certainly can provide insight into the mechanisms underlying the "how" of the disease process, but they cannot always provide the "why" underlying or initiating the sequence of biological events. Context frequently provides the "why," whereas biology frequently provides the "how," though these distinctions do not hold strictly.

Two aspects of context should be differentiated. The first one is contemporaneous and the second historical. Say a six-year-old injures his fingers in closing his father's car door. The contemporary context is father, car door closing, and boy's fingers in door. The historical context could be illustrated in this case by an earlier argument between father and son about appropriate dress for the day's outing. The more remote historical context might be a divorced father after a long absence wanting to make the outing a success. Adequate understanding of the "cause" of the injury and its treatment and future prevention requires in addition to understanding the pathology of injury knowledge of contemporary and historical contexts.

Underlying this discussion of context is the proposition of requiring the consideration of "multifactorial" elements in accounting for the expression of pathology. Even in the almost purely genetically derived disease of Huntington's Chorea, there are interactions among genes that modify the degree of disability in patients. More often than not, the "multifactorial" influences of behavioral, psychological, and social contexts are important factors in accounting for the etiology, maintenance, and expression of the disease process. Therefore knowledge of behavioral and social sciences becomes essential in understanding the "why" along with understanding the "how" of clinical medicine.

Fortunately today the education and training of physicians goes beyond the narrow psychosocial paradigms of fifty years ago: the family and the doctor–patient relationship. In my view these two contexts, although important, are inadequate to understanding context in the broader sense. The importance of multiple contexts is still neglected today in medical schools and residency programs. I submit that social and behavioral scientists (including historians) are in a good position to sensitize physicians to the contextual facet in understanding patients and their illnesses. Ideally the social and behavioral sciences relevant to medicine should be part of every medical student's education while in medical school.

If evaluating patients from a contextual point of view proves helpful to practicing physicians, it might be possible for physicians to insist on additional time to collect information from patients, using the "context" of the patients' problems to understand the "why" and inform the "how" in the treatment. More importantly, the contextual perspective may provide insight for a scientific basis for prevention, a relatively neglected concern in current medical practice.

A Point of View: Medical Care for the 21st Century

*"One of the essential qualities of the clinician
is the interest in humanity, for the secret of the care
of the patient is in caring for the patient."*
—Francis Weld Peabody (1902)

*"When you care for yourself you are being cared for by
someone who really cares."*
—Garrison Keillor, humorist on National Public Radio
commenting on American Medicine (2004)

The Political/Economic Context of American Medical Care: My discussion of the American health care system will necessarily be truncated since this is not the central focus of this essay. However, I will take the opportunity as a member of HMS '53 to present my views if only to stimulate discussion and provide some evidence for the variety in the views of members of my class.

I begin with the assumption that it is in the national as well as in the individual interest to have available a system of medical services for the maintenance of health, the diagnosis and treatment of disease, and rehabilitation for return to the community. That we do not have such a system currently in the United States is easily demonstrated by public health statistics, personal anecdotes of dissatisfied consumers and unhappy health care personnel, and comparisons with medical systems in other advanced countries.

My focus will be on the deficiencies in the current system with only brief attention to the allocation of resources within the health care system, a vast subject owned by the growth industry of health care economics. I will organize my discussion around concepts introduced by my Stanford colleague, economist Professor Victor Fuchs on the goals of a health care systems. In addition to his four goals—fairness, efficiency, democracy, freedom—I will add a fifth goal of security (i.e., trust), a goal of central importance to patients experiencing the threat of illness.

Fairness: The single most critical deficiency in American medicine is the absence of easily accessed affordable services for lower-income individuals. Forty-three million individuals, probably a low estimate, are reported to be without health insurance. There are vast discrepancies between the care provided for those in the lowest quartile of the economic scale and those in the highest quartile. While new cathedrals for medical services have been constructed for the favored few, decrepit community health centers are provided for the many. All too frequently, those of low income defer health care until a crisis intervenes, and then they seek expensive emergency care, if available, adding to the burden of cost of medical services. Even when public resources are available, waiting times are long, distance to health centers great, and individual attention non-existent.

A second aspect of unfairness in the current system is tying the insurance coverage for medical services to the place of employment. Such a system might be fair under conditions of full employment, or portability of coverage with changes of employment. The ability of small businesses to afford insurance coverage is considerably lower than it is for the larger companies, frequently leading to little or no coverage of employees by the smaller firms.

Efficiency: The lack of systematic relationships between community health centers, practicing physicians, regional hospitals, and tertiary care centers is a major loss for institutions, caretaking personnel and patients' care. The absence of information flow from the periphery reduces the chance for excellent diagnoses and treatment, and subsequent rehabilitation without costly duplication of diagnostic testing.

A second deficiency is the inadequate communication system among health personnel in various departments of the Hospital. The lack of easily recordable, reliable information on patients' status sets the stage for poor treatment and error in patient care. Computer technology can provide for each patient in a web page type, recording information that could be easily transported to caretakers outside the hospital in summary form, thereby reducing error and avoiding costly duplication.

Freedom: Implied in the goal of freedom is the crucial element of *choice* and exit for patients and sometimes for physicians. The simple fee-for-service system, a quaint relic of the past except in boutique medical practice, provided maximum opportunity for freedom. In the current scene there are considerable restrictions of choice, and very little possibility of exit as anyone who has attempted to change physicians or get a second opinion under the HMO system can attest. If there is to be more than an illusion of choice, patients must be educated about the realistic possibilities for treatment including the opportunity for a second opinion. Because information on "competencies" of physicians and norms of practice, are difficult for the typical patient to acquire, proactive guidance by heath professionals should be part of the routine practice of medicine.

Democracy: The absence of democracy in the medical care system, that is input from consumers, employees, and professionals into the administration of the system, is a major deficit. Medicine has a long history of being part of a hierarchical culture, perhaps defensible in the past, when physicians had direct contact with their patients. Doctors came to know their patients and patients to know their doctors establishing more collegial relationships over time. In current circumstances with more attenuated relationships by physicians and distant relationships of administrators, hierarchical systems are not productive of patient satisfaction and trust, even more so in the presence of the opaque organizational structures which seem to the current norm. Since uncertainty is detrimental to high morale for professionals, patients, and staff. Opening up the system to closer scrutiny may have a salutary effect for everyone, especially for the patient. My proposal would be representation on Boards of Directors of corporate and non-corporate providers of health services to practicing doctors, nurses, consumers, and staff complementing the representation from the financial, legal and business communities. Perhaps contact from a variety of individuals on these boards could produce a better system, at least one deserving of more trust than currently exists.

Trust and Security: Trust in the medical system and in a personal physician is an essential ingredient for promotion of health and recovery from illness and disability. The uncertainty built into the current system through absence of integrated health planning, the worry about affordability when illness occurs, and suspicion about conflict of interest in caretakers, leads to a profound lack of trust by patients, ultimately affecting their recovery. Patients require assurance that caretakers are acting in their best interest—that physicians and their associates are advocates for them and not for some amorphous corporate entity far removed from their immediate concerns. At the time of crisis patients are not interested in the choices they could have made in the past, but are intensely concerned that the current choice

be the best one under the circumstances, the standard for judgment being "Can I trust this person to act on my behalf?"

A Possible Solution: Having briefly presented my list of problems
besetting the current medical care system, it behooves me to
provide the reader with my fantasies about a system that might
address these problems and possibly have a chance for implementation over the next generation.

Community health centers should be the first contact for anyone who requires medical services. The housing and cost of professional staff—doctors, nurses, social workers, and medical
assistants—should be borne by the county, state, and federal system through taxes earmarked as the government's contribution
for support of a crucial portion of the social infrastructure. These
primary facilities would not be part of the market system, because
the market system at this level has been shown to be incomplete,
inappropriate, expensive, notoriously inefficient, and frequently
not available to the communities most in need of services.

Beyond the community health center, I envision a regional
health care level of service where market forces might be appropriate, though my hunch is that they would have to be supplemented by subsidies for areas with low appeal for private market
forces. These regional centers should have a multipractice service, including surgical, medical, orthopedic, neurological, and
psychological/psychiatric services as well as rehabilitation services. They would maintain a coordinated, computerized record
system for themselves, the community health centers, and tertiary care hospitals providing more specialized services would be
available. The record system should be arranged so that personal
information would be secure, but the "public" information
regarding demographics, illness, and treatment would be available for clinical research. The data from all patients would provide oversight regarding care and treatment as well as
demographic information. Collated information in sufficient
detail for clinical use on disease outbreaks, unusual patient reactions to medications and traumas, would be as readily available
on a weekly basis for the field of medicine, as are the daily
weather reports for the airline and transportation industry

The organizational schema would be such that regional medical centers would be responsible for the standards of the community system. The community system would be associated with

the regional system, and the regional system would be available for education and consultation. Physicians as educators would then compete with pharmaceutical company representatives to present scientifically based practice of medicine and advise practitioners on medication usage. The fee-for-service, private practice system might be parallel to or associated with this proposed system, or operate outside of it with a private insurance system, but nonetheless would participate in clinical research activities.

The current tertiary care university research center hospitals do well in medical student resident and fellowship education, and extremely well in clinical and basic research, but are more problematic when delivering service across departmental specialties and to professionals practicing outside of the hospital. However, the coordination and systematization of information between and among specialties taking care of a patient within the same hospital needs considerable improvement, and requires vast improvement in communication with outside clinics, non-hospital doctors, and rehabilitation centers.

Financing the System: This is not the place, nor do I have the competence, to deliver a detailed economic and political analysis of the problem. In participating in this volume of opinions, representing a spectrum of viewpoints of the HMS '53, after fifty years in a medical career, I will briefly present my views, likely shared by some classmates and certainly disagreed with by many others.

There are numerous examples—some good, some indifferent—among the industrial nations of the Western world of possible systems. I propose serious examination of other systems for ideas and models that might be applicable to at least some portion of our current "jerry-rigged" non-system. I particularly recommend examining the Canadian system (administrative costs 8%–12%) for some of its practices. The British, German, and Scandinavian systems also might provide some ideas. Regardless of whether or not any of these approaches prove applicable to the United States case (administrative costs 24%–26%), they suggest possible empirical tests of systems, varying by state, or region of our country. The important point I wish to make is that the delivery of medical services should be a part of the basic social infrastructure of our country, along with education, transportation, public safety, shelter, nutrition, and personal security.

This basic human right might be served in part through the private sector, but chiefly would be supported by funds derived from the public sector, fully supported by the tax system. These public funds should be derived from a progressive tax, where those at the top of the economic scale contribute more and those at the bottom contribute less. All residents should be involved in contributing financially as part of their duty in fulfilling obligations of citizenship and residence in the society.

I remain skeptical about the ability of the private sector to provide services using market forces alone, especially for those at the lower end of the socio-economic scale. We have tested this approach and it has failed, with the results of inadequate services, unhappy professional personnel, and large groups not served, along with high administrative costs. I believe we should provide true universal coverage independent of employment, paid for by mandatory taxes on private corporations and by taxes on the individual as part of the public, supplemented by personal insurance for those who opt only for a private system. This program should be placed on an actuarially sound basis, not subject to annual political manipulation. Individuals would have a choice of services—paid for at a minimum level determined by the public system. Services generally would be obtained in excellent public institutions, but also could be obtained in mixed public/private institutions, or purely private institutions for those who prefer that route.

Regardless of whether any given individual uses the public service or private system, all will contribute to the cost of the public system on a progressive basis with no cap on the amount of income to be taxed, and no differential based on whether income is derived from employment, from capital gains, or from dividends earned in the United States or Internationally.

Clearly this proposed single-payer schema will involve considerable financing. The public, including non-paying citizens and residents at the bottom of the economic scale who do not vote but should do so, and those citizens at the top of the economic scale who vote but do not pay their fair share of the cost, should be informed that the proposed plan is the price that all must pay for living in a complex, interrelated political, social, and economic system in the 21st century. This rational system for delivery of medical services, despite the trenchant comment of Garrison Keillor in 2004 may yet enable us to achieve the 1902 goals of Dr. Peabody: ". . . an interest in humanity, for the secret of the care of the patient is in caring for the patient." It is the minimum legacy we should leave for the next generations.

The Context for the Promotion of Health

Planfulness and Prevention Versus the "Free Market": Given the bio- psycho- socio-cultural perspective guiding my work, I will present what I believe to be a reasonable approach to promotion of health and medical care appropriate for all the citizens of our country and ultimately for all societies that do not as yet have minimal services for their citizens. Much of what I write is not original, and much of what I recommend is provided in many countries—for example, in Canada—and in many countries of northwestern and central Europe. That my proposals are not current practice in the United States still amazes me. I will not be so bold or foolish as to speculate here on the reasons why we cannot catch up to other modern societies in providing health care and medical services, but my recommendations for improvements may hint at some of the impediments.

First, health care information should be universally available, at the very least beginning with middle school and high school students with the purpose of reducing the effects of disease and illness, directly and indirectly the promotion of positive health habits. Prevention of illnesses such as diabetes, and cardiovascular diseases through diet and proper physical activity would more than pay for itself in the long run by reducing disability from stroke, heart attack, and arthritis later on in adulthood.

Second, information about how the medical system really operates should be available for adolescents and young adults, so that future discussions about the positive and negative aspects of the system can be intelligently addressed. In this way there may be an opportunity for making changes in the system from the "bottom-up."

Third, turning to the behavioral, psychological, and psychiatric realms, I propose the active promotion of healthy intrauterine environments, positive mother–infant attachment, social bonding within the family in early childhood, fostering of positive peer relationships, and provision of structured and stimulating environments at least through age six as the minimum to ensure socially and cognitively competent children, who will be able to accept the challenges of an education leading toward an autonomous, considerate, and competent adulthood.

Here I wish to state a case for social and behavioral scientists, in addition to economists, to become involved in research on problems confronting current American medical practice. I believe social and behavioral scientists are uniquely equipped to study the social psychological aspects of institutional and small group organization, the cognitive psychology of communication, the biopsychology of stress, the developmental implications of childhood, adolescence, youth, adulthood, and the aged on disease processes, and as well the motivational circumstances favoring or inhibiting rehabilitation after illness.

If one accepts this argument about the importance of prevention of disease and the promotion of positive social and psychological development in the earliest years, then we might consider how market forces might encourage physicians (and other health professionals) to enter the fields most relevant to prevention of disease and promotion of psychosocial development. To no one's surprise, physician remuneration by subspecialty is inversely related to the distance of relevancy to prevention and developmental and psychosocial concerns. Pay is lowest for pediatrics, psychiatry, social medicine, and public health, and highest for subspecialties least involved in prevention, that is, general surgery, anesthesiology, radiology, and plastic surgery. The medical profession has not sufficiently addressed the potential of cost reduction of medical care through prevention and promotion of positive psychosocial development in the child's earliest years.

Behind the suggestions I have proposed is my skepticism about the "mindless marketplace" correcting these deficiencies. I believe that leaders in medicine and the social sciences should speak out about medical and psychosocial issues where they are really expert, and when not expert to call on others to help them toward the goal of safe, affordable, and efficient medical care, ignoring the current worship of medical administrators at the temple of the "free market."

The discussion of some of these suggestions likely will take years to work through, and one or two generations of political activity to implement. This assumes, of course, there is sufficient time to do so in this age of suicidal bombers, domestic and foreign. However, starting now is probably worth the effort, since looking skyward for danger from incoming enemy missiles, listening to the more dangerous missals spewing forth from the airwaves, while ignoring the most dangerous threats here on earth—gnorance, poverty, and poor health—is surely ironic if not downright insane.

The Contemporary Context: Between unmanaged care and non–free-market medicine we have a financial, social, and medical disaster on our hands in the United States. The high cost of services, the non-availability of services to many urban and most rural residents, the inadequate training of physicians, nurses, and other medical personnel for 21st-century practice and the absence of planning for wellness rather than for illness are merely a sample of critical issues. The political system, beset by the usual pressure from groups who have a stake in keeping the present system intact, does not respond to local and national need. Our national leaders use diversionary tactics, relegating health issues to the realm of personal irresponsibility, as if responsibility could mend a badly flawed system.

Hortatory language about individual planfulness and responsibility is particularly odious when our national leadership is embarked on a war without planful and responsible consideration of its non-military aftermath. Non-planful and non-responsible leadership in health matters has demonstrably failed to work in mending or replacing our current inadequate system. Apart from equity issues, our survival as a nation in a period of international crisis demands responsible and planful leadership from medical and health professionals, as we can no longer depend on the political leadership to solve this critical problem in our society.

Finale

I shall not leave this valedictory essay without commenting on the great advances made in our society over the course of my lifetime. I began with memories of the Economic Depression of 1929–37, the Midwest Dust Bowl, the urban unemployed, the brutal treatment of African Americans, the covert and sometimes overt anti-Semitism I personally experienced. My narrative continues with the crossing of the great divide in my life, World War II—for me, the *Great War*—where I matured, was given responsibilities in furthering a noble cause, and was thankful for surviving when two of my closest friends did not. Our government then was not merely satisfied with winning the war but also prepared for the peace, at least in Europe with the Marshall Plan and at home with the GI Bill and other social programs to manage a transition to the future with an aura of hope. African-Americans were given greater respect by integration of the military. Jews were no longer despised, possibly because of the Holocaust in Europe, possibly because of establishment of the State of Israel. Elite educational institutions were rethinking exclusion of unwanted minorities. The country was moving toward acceptance of diversity and toward inclusionary rather than exclusionary values.

This ideal has continued steadily, albeit slowly, to the present. Women are accepted for positions of leadership in medicine, law, education, business, and politics. African-Americans are finally beginning to develop a solid middle and upper class, essential for acceptance in our "classless society," though far too many are still in the underclass. East Asian and South Asian migration, along with Mestizos, Hispanics, Middle Eastern Arabs and Jews, have filled in the color gradient. We can no longer maintain the fiction that Americans are only pleasantly pinkish White or beautifully Black—now we clearly see people in enticing shades of red, yellow, and brown. Simple crude racism is now almost impossible to express aloud, though subtle non-verbal racism still exists. Where we fail now is our avoidance of discussion of social class. Here the elites (economic, political, and social) and the lower classes agree: "We will not discuss this issue because, really aren't we all middle-class?" I would like our political leadership to recognize the reality of social class differences, and confront the economic inequalities that exist head-on, so that all members of our society might prosper, health included, because then they could face this very great danger to our national well-being in the 21st Century.

Dr. Leiderman remained in Boston after medical school, training in neurology and psychiatry. He then served as a research faculty member at HMS. Called to Stanford as an Associate Professor, Dr. Leiderman remained there for forty-two years. He has traveled widely on work related projects, and has also been honored with a Guggenheim Fellowship, and fellowships at the Center for Advanced Study in Behavioral Sciences and at the Rockefeller Center, Bellagio, Lake Como, Italy.

Miscellaneous Musings

Is It Ever Too Late to Change Your Mind?

Frederik C. Hansen

In a busy practice it is often easiest for one to "go along to get along." However, in retirement there is time to be more skeptical of long accepted perspectives of life's problems and one's future plans. The following are some revisionist views that are displacing some of my long held opinions. I only wish that I had the writing and thinking skills to frame them in more convincing terms, but they are an illustrative sampling of my re-contemplation of these views.

As I circle life's drain, I am spending much effort on getting my life in order. My workshop is now in first class shape with all of the tools and materials in neat array. My desk is headed in that direction, and I am even thinking of putting a fifty-year marriage's worth of photographs in order. (If only I had put names and dates on them when they came back from the developer!)

Similarly, I have been revamping some of the accepted truths that I bought into and some of the plans that I made without due thought. What follows are some of my life's end thoughts and plans that depart considerably from my past expectations.

Has Any Prohibition Ever Worked as Intended?

By definition crimes can't exist without a prohibition. To be successful, a professional criminal needs a crime that is profitable, and profitability increases in proportion to the risk involved, just as it does in the financial markets. Murder, mayhem, fraud and extortion do not follow the rules of the marketplace in quite the way that illicit trade in prohibited substances does.

The trade in prohibited drugs is exceedingly profitable, largely because of legal prohibitions. Tough drug laws and their enforcement serve only to raise the value of these substances. The drug lords benefit from stringent laws with weak enforcement. The

197

cops can't find the dealers, but the users have no such problem. This filthy traffic is soiling everyone along the line—from the growers in the third world countries, through the transporters, the dealers, the users, and far too many innocent bystanders.

The situation is hopeless unless we can take the profits away. The scum of society runs an efficient, lucrative and ruthlessly violent industry to service user demand. The huge profits allow unscrupulous dealers to buy their way into legitimate businesses where scrupulousness seems already in short supply. Properly paid off politicians can look tough on crime while playing into the hands of the dealers with unenforceable laws.

The marketing of habituating drugs is well illustrated in the tobacco industry, while the criminal aspects for alcohol were well illustrated during what we rightly called "Prohibition."

Alcohol, tobacco, drugs, greasy food, gun ownership, sexually transmitted diseases, aggressive driving, and laziness are all personal choices that are best controlled by education, taxation, and example. Let those of us who have chosen to avoid them (well, most of them) get on with our lives without becoming innocent victims of the crimes associated with the prohibition of drugs. Didn't we learn that once before? Are any of you as tired of having your house burglarized and your car ripped off as I am? Take the profits out of drug prohibition. Decriminalize most drugs; control their quality and sales as with alcohol; severely penalize intoxicated behavior; tax drugs heavily to support education and addict rehabilitation; reform rather than criminalize their management, as with all the other deadly choices we must make in our lives.

Drugs have been only marginal in my life and practice, so I know this sounds foolishly naive to those of you who have gained more expertise from confronting drugs in your clinical practices or your family life. But, on the other hand, where has a century of such expertise gotten us? Prohibitions have never worked in the past and there is little reason to believe that will change in the future.

Lifestyle—I Never Knew I Had One

I learned during a year on the bench in freshman football that if you have not been out there learning to struggle on the soccer field in grade school, and if you lack the killer instinct to win, you couldn't suddenly acquire it in high school. Coaches are generally there to win, not to teach those who lack natural ability. Schools may have remedial reading and math classes, but they do not have remedial athletics for the clumsy.

By middle age I harvested the yield of my sloth, and after my first bypass, began biking and jogging, and eating the right foods, if there can be such. The result for my children was that, while they did not become super athletes, they all have acquired good eating and exercise habits. They know what may lurk in their genes. Many young families now realize that it is their responsibility to teach their children the importance of lifelong regular physical activity as the spine of a healthy lifestyle.

I now realize in my penultimate years that continued exercise of mind and body may forestall the inevitable. If I ever develop an urge to be tattooed it will say: Do Not Resuscitate! I have no desire to live if my headquarters are shut down. Fitness appropriate for age is a gift to be strived for.

Bodily Changes

As I was growing up I was constantly amazed by the changes that were occurring in my body, and I generally looked with pleasant anticipation for what was coming next. Now as a superannuated adult who is growing down, the changes in my body are still quite interesting but the sense of pleasant anticipation is greatly diminished. I am in no hurry for the next changes to occur.

A Dog's Life

To survive, all of the animals of God's world must have a strategy to survive the growing encroachments of mankind. They must avoid us, fight us, feed us, clothe us, serve us, protect us, amuse us, or in some other ways escape our often-destructive influences.

Our relationship with the haughty cat is somewhat conditional and leaves us with a rather one-sided affection dependent on our providing food and shelter in return for more distant expressions of affection. Certainly their ability to control the rodent encroachment on our food supplies was a major factor in the development of the relationship, especially while our agrarian ancestors were extremely dependent on protecting their supplies of seeds through the dormant season. Feral cats generally lead a more solitary existence even where they exist in large numbers. You can usually own a dog, but a cat must own you or there is no relationship. I have found the relationships with dog and cat to be very different.

When first married, my wife and I had two lovely Siamese cats to which we developed strong emotional attachments and severe allergies. It was a sad day indeed when we shipped them off to a new home with some dear friends. No one knew then of the strong antigens in their saliva.

The survival ploy that has meant the most to me has been that of the dog, who probably went from the pack hunter, to the hunted, to the hunting companion, protector, and the source of much unconditional love for his master. Where else can you find that? My lifetime of ten dogs has included: a Belgian Shepherd, a Doberman Pinscher, a German Shepherd, four Labrador Retrievers, a Great Dane, and two mixed terriers.

In retirement I have tried to find some satisfaction in volunteering as a dog walker for the SPCA and in working with several hundred rescued animals. I have been impressed by the ability of even the most cruelly treated animals to recover their ability to join the human pack and become loving companions. This re-socialization of animals coming from extremely wretched circumstances is a most rewarding aspect of volunteering and of the rescue and adoption process. They do not seem to carry into a new relationship the heavy emotional load that the abused human child does.

Closing the Loop

As always in medicine there are differences of opinion regarding the value of dissection as a means of learning anatomy, but I fall decidedly on the side that feels that this experience is essential— even for the non-surgeons. At a minimum, there is the real anatomy, starkly and accurately laid out before your eyes and touch. Individual variations lurk to trap those who place undue trust in the anatomy books of Gray and Grant. A cadaver remains little more than the hulk of the person who wore that body in life. On the dissection table there are none of the vibrant physiological processes that pumped life and spirit into it. That experience awaited us in our clinical years.

Because I personally see eternal life only in terms of the DNA that passes on to one's offspring, not to any belief in heaven, the soul, or the hereafter, I have determined that I will complete the loop so to speak, and gift my cadaver to the Harvard Medical School or to The Johns Hopkins Anatomy Department (the development offices have a more substantial gift in mind, I am sure). It is my fervent hope that the dissection team that descends on my remains will not be misled by any abnormalities that I may harbor and that my circuitry will serve them well in evaluating the intact patients they encounter in their future endeavors. If there should prove to be life after death, that could prove to be a most interesting experience and I promise to keep you posted if there be heavenly or hellish e-mail.

A Malapproach to Malpractice

Remember the good old days when they had flight insurance vending machines in the airport and for a few quarters you could buy a $100,000 policy for your round trip? It had several virtues: the vendors made money; the passenger was insured against risk; malfeasance did not have to be proven. Over and above those things it drove home to the passengers that they were taking a risk—which fact probably had much to do with its failure as a business venture.

Medical misadventures are not as clear cut as a plane crash, but bad results come about in many ways. The physician knowingly did something wrong, the physician unknowingly did something wrong, the physician did nothing wrong but there was a bad outcome, the patient did something wrong, a secondary condition caused a bad outcome, or the gods of chance did something wrong.

Whatever the cause of a bad outcome or a perceived bad outcome, the modern patient is being educated to seek redress in court. Practitioners are partially responsible for this because of their unwillingness long ago to buy into a no-fault system of risk sharing.

The problem is that there is no way of compensating the patient who, through no fault of the caregivers or his own, becomes severely injured or disabled following treatment. Juries see only the bad result that may blind them to the quality of care that preceded that result.

There will always be malpractice that must be dealt with as such, but there should be a no-fault system of compensation for the patient who has a bad outcome through no one's fault. This would relieve much of the burden of malpractice settlements that have no basis in malpractice. My decision to retire after forty years of practice was partially because I had escaped any claims of malpractice though I had certainly had my share of bad outcomes.

Grounding the Third Rail

At the time of the class of 53's fiftieth reunion we were asked to expound on some subjects of pleasure or pain in our lives since graduation. Many responded and those responses became the seed that grew in Fritz Loewenstein's mind into this collection of essays. Buried in that anniversary collection was a remarkable heartfelt statement by one of our classmates who committed the unpardonable: he touched the third rail of politics—Israel and Palestine. He asked why so few prominent Jews had publicly denounced the unpardonable actions between Israel and the Palestinians?

I grew up in the Pacific Northwest in relative innocence of either Arab or Jew and it was not until medical school and my subsequent training and practice that I was fortunate enough to acquire many Arab and Jewish friends. One of my junior associates in practice was a Palestinian who made me aware of the flourishing culture that Arabs had attained during the Dark Ages of western culture, only to fall into self-destructive conflicts and regressive cultural and religious practices that impeded further progressive development.

When I told one of my cynical Jewish friends that I thought C. P. Snow was correct in saying that the Diaspora had bred a superior group of people, he replied that I just hadn't met enough of them yet. In my limited experience, however, no other group of people have been in leadership roles in such great numbers on moral, ethical, philosophical, and scientific issues as the Jews. Why then are they sitting by and watching as the festering war with the Palestinians drags the world down into utter chaos?

The main organized Jewish movement against the war is through the likes of Neturei Karta, which has been primarily against Zionism and only secondarily against the mistreatment of the Palestinians. From time immemorial the Middle East has been a site of constant turmoil triangulated between the Muslims, the Jews and the Christians.

Time seems to be bearing out the statement that "War Is Not The Answer."

The recent experiences in Rwanda and South Africa with "Truth and Reconciliation" offer interesting examples of the strategy of confession and the tactic of forgiveness as a way of circumventing the ceaseless feuding conflict that follows reciprocating acts of retribution. Perhaps it is time for the fundamentalists to practice those aspects of their religions that deal with forgiveness as a strategy and a tactic. Wouldn't it be the Christian/Jewish/Muslim thing to do? My reading of the New and Old Testaments and the Koran disclose perfectly good arguments for this as well as those worn-out arguments for bloody retribution that continue to plague us. We should avoid the mistake of confusing religious beliefs, passions, and myths with common sense.

Speaking of Common Sense

Dr. Thomas Turner was Dean of The Johns Hopkins Medical School, 1957–1968. He died at age 100 in September 2002. Enclosed in his Christmas card for 1993 was the following:

"A Few Things Learned During A Long Life

"Date what you write. Otherwise, neither you nor anyone else will likely remember whether it was written months or years ago. (Of course, no one may care.)

"Almost all soups can be improved by a dash of sherry.

"The quality of life and the effort to improve it are what it's all about.

"When given a book, thank the giver within forty-eight hours; otherwise you really will have to read it.

"Love, affection and compassion are allied, but not the same. Reciprocated love is rare; cherish and guard it well. Affection supports life's infrastructures; compassion underpins the world.

"Hold on to the banisters going down stairs."

To such wisdom I can only add for my surgeon friends: Always take a pre-op photograph—you never know when you may get a good result!

Addendum: Since these rambling thoughts were submitted, many fate-filled events have occurred. They bring to mind the following:

When my parents were in their elder years they felt that they had been blessed to overcome their parents' very humble circumstances enabling them to see their son become the first and only college graduate in the family. They also saw the world as becoming an increasingly dangerous place and, while they had been fortunate to have lived in what they termed a "golden era," after the 1960s they despaired of the state of the world they were leaving to their children and grandchildren.My wife and I, in turn, feel blessed to have exceeded our parents' humble circumstances, and have been able to see all of our children and all of our grandchildren on track to complete college. We most truly appreciate the good fortune that our happy family has enjoyed. We have been able to live during a "golden era," and yet we despair of the sometimes-wretched state of the world that will be our childrens' and grandchildrens' to navigate.

So perhaps we all just delude ourselves into the Panglossian thinking that we each lived in a best of all possible worlds that is soon destined to go into the tank. Mr. Bush has certainly proved that unintelligent design should be debated.

Dr. Hansen was born in Tacoma, Washington, in 1926, became board certified in General and Plastic Surgery, and engaged in private practice thereof in Baltimore, Maryland, from 1960 to 1990. In retirement he is most proud of his wife, four children and eight grandchildren. He should be able to shoot his age in golf—if he lives to be ninety.

An Atheist Examines Monotheism

Philip Bromberg

Having grown up in the United States as a Jewish atheist during the time of what is now called the "Holocaust," and later become a physician and a scientist, I have attempted to describe the relationship of religious dogma to anti-Semitism and to some aspects of science and medicine. One might also examine the relation of monotheism and its interpreters to Islamic fundamentalism and world terrorism, which have forced themselves on our unwilling attention, but I have chosen to leave that problem aside.

Anti-Semitism: Anti-Semitism has been an important force in much of the world for over two thousand years. The decline and dissolution of the independent Hebrew state following its meteoric rise under Saul, David, and Solomon, leading to the first destruction of the Temple and to captivity in Babylon, and later to the destruction of the second Temple by the Romans, did not prevent or mitigate hatred of the Jews. Perhaps it was even intensified by the Diaspora as Jews migrated throughout the Roman world. Hundreds of years later, Jews migrated throughout the Islamic world as Muslim Arabs conquered the Middle East and North Africa and moved up through the Iberian peninsula into southern France where their surge was finally halted at the battle of Poitiers.

Although Judaism is the oldest of the three monotheistic religions and is the root from which Christianity arose, Jews have never been particularly numerous. And unlike Christianity and Islam, which actively convert heathens and infidels, Judaism keeps itself aloof. When organized Judaism of the time turned away from the new religion and did not recognize Jesus as the Messiah, it became the enemy. The gospels, written decades after the death of Jesus, himself a Jew, are overtly anti-Semitic.

I don't know exactly why Islam is anti-Semitic as well, but it has been so since the time of the Prophet himself who authorized the massacre of two Hebrew tribes in Arabia. Perhaps it is because, like the Jews, Muslims claim their roots from Abraham (through Hagar and Ishmael rather than Sarah and Isaac) and because, in the Book of Genesis, God is said to have promised land and protection in the Near East to Abraham and his descendants. The notion of the return of a Jewish state to the "promised land" is anathema to the Arabs. That is why I am profoundly pessimistic about the future of Israel in the Arab sea, and why advising Israel to trade land for peace is not going to help Israel to survive.

Europe and the Americas have been dominated by Christianity, which has persecuted the Jews for about two thousand years. The suffering and torture of Jesus before and during the crucifixion is ascribed to the Jews and their religious leaders by Matthew, though not as explicitly as in the other gospels. Christian teaching and preaching has put Christ's blood squarely on the heads of the Jews and their descendants. Medieval "passion" plays re-enacting the crucifixion of Jesus and surrounding events have always excited hatred of Jews among the audiences and frequently led to assault upon and murder of Jews.

When I was growing up in the 1930s in a non-Jewish lower middle class neighborhood in Queens Village, New York, I was routinely shoved around and beaten up on my five-block walk to and from Public School 109. I asked two friends who lived next door why I was singled out for such treatment and learned that they were taught in Sunday school that the Jews had killed Christ and were therefore culpable of an inexpiable sin.

In the 1930s Queens Village was a hotbed of pro-German, pro-Nazi sentiment and the Silvershirts and Brownshirts (modeled on their Nazi counterparts) marched and manifested about a mile from my house. Of course, Father Coughlin's anti-Semitic diatribes on the radio were a staple of the intellectual diet.

The Holocaust was beginning in Europe but it took a few years for the Germans to move from "legal" deprivation of the civil rights and status in society of Jews to the brutality toward and dehumanization of Jews that converted them into a subhuman species fit for organized extermination. This was of course the policy known as the "final solution." Six million Jewish men, women and children were systematically hunted down and murdered in just a few years. And the Germans found enthusiastic support for their policy in most European countries, I am sad to say. (Denmark was an outstanding exception.) Nor did the United States open its borders to European Jews as political refugees in mortal danger despite them being largely educated and productive people.

I suppose it was the (brief) period of Western guilt feelings about the Holocaust plus President Harry Truman's determination that brought about the creation (re-creation) of the state of Israel in 1947. And, quite miraculously, the new state survived the military attack of all the neighboring Arab states. Israel has continued to defend itself successfully against further attacks, but of course its first defeat would be its last, with an ensuing massacre of millions of Jews by the Arabs while the world expresses its "regrets" but does nothing. Israel is not a fully secular state. But in spite of this handicap and being perpetually on a war footing and living in an area with minimal resources, it is the only democracy in the region and has accomplished prodigious feats in science, technology and agriculture while resettling millions of immigrants.

Here in the post-war United States anti-Semitism seemed to gradually diminish, although there are still plenty of "discriminating" clubs, residential areas, banks, etc. When I applied to twenty medical schools in 1948, with an outstanding scholastic record, I was turned down by all the New York City schools, all of which had very small Jewish quotas. But Harvard (after considerable hesitation and multiple interviews, probably due to my youth) offered me first a place on its waiting list and then a place in the class of '53. (I've always had the notion that it was my interview with Professor Christian Anfinsen, later a Nobel laureate, during which the conversation turned to chamber music, that tipped the balance in my favor, because Professor Anfinsen was an enthusiastic amateur violist and playing violin and viola had been, and still is, an important part of my life.) When I arrived at Harvard Medical School in September, 1949, I was astonished to note that—judging from family names—about one third of my 110 classmates were Jewish although there were only seven women and two African-Americans. There were relatively few Jewish professors apart from those at the Beth Israel Hospital, but that situation was to change rapidly as well.

Jews have intermarried extensively with non-Jews and now generally feel integrated and accepted in the United States. But that was also true of Germany in the 1930s and we know what happened there. More concretely, since the death of Martin Luther King in 1968, we have seen the emergence of unabashed anti-Semitism among blacks leavened with a dash of Islam. And as I write, the anti-Semitic film "The Passion of the Christ" has been released. The producer/director, Mel Gibson, has outdone all the feeble efforts of previous passion plays, portraying the Jews as well as their religious leaders as screaming for the blood of Jesus, overcoming Pilate's feeble resistance and then physically assaulting Jesus in the most horrific manner that modern cinematographic technology can provide. The film appears to have raised little or no moral opposition among Christians. I've not heard of protests by Christian leaders, and notably among Catholics (despite the move away from the blanket condemnation of the Jews at Vatican II 40 years ago). Gibson himself is a Catholic of the more reactionary variety who presumably does not accept the results of Vatican II and Gibson's father is said to be a Holocaust-denier.

There are lots of angry zealots in our midst and a film like this is perfectly capable of convincing them that they should be killing Jews: indeed that it is a highly moral thing to do.

In Europe after World War II very few Jews had survived in the countries of central Europe, so overt anti-Semitism became more difficult to practice at home. But the state of Israel furnishes a convenient target for anti-Semitism. Jews can be attacked not as Jews but as a political entity, and the Arabs are there to do the dirty work. In Soviet Russia, anti-Semitism remained alive and well after the Bolshevik Revolution despite the official atheism of Soviet state and the presence of people of Jewish origin (e.g., Trotsky, Litvinov, Kaganovich) at high levels in the government, in the arts (e.g., Babel, Akhmatova), and in science (e.g., Landau and many others). Many Russian Jews have emigrated since the frontiers were opened in the past two decades. Turning to western Europe, anti-Semitism is very much alive and well in France where it has always been a factor despite the separation of church and state by Napoleon Bonaparte and the fact that France has even had Jewish prime ministers (Léon Blum before World War II, Pierre Mendès-France during the Indo-China peace negotiation, and Laurent Fabius briefly about a decade ago). And France's large and growing Muslim population (now exceding 10%) doesn't help that situation. In Britain we recently had the example of the Nuffield Professor of Pathology at Oxford who refused to accept a well-qualified Israeli post-doctorate in his laboratory because the young man had served in the Israel Defense Force. In Islamic countries it is extremely dangerous to be a Jew. The fact he was Jewish surely played a role when the reporter Danny Pearl was abducted and murdered in Pakistan. There are probably no more than a handful of Jews still living in the entire Arab–Muslim world. After World War II, most emigrated to Israel.

It is interesting that China has avoided religious domination for many centuries and that Confucianism remains at the root of the Chinese social order. The "golden rule" in its negative Confucian form is an important precept: "Do not unto others what you would not have done unto you." Respect for education and learning, and for teachers, are other elements that are remarkably similar to Jewish ethics.

What is truly remarkable is that such a small number of people are able to excite so much anger and malice. From an ecological standpoint the 10–15 million people who constitute world Jewry would be classified as an endangered species! By contrast there are literally billions of Christians and Muslims. Of course these 10–15 million Jews are concentrated in the United States and other countries in North and South America, in Israel, and in Western Europe—whose total population must be of the order of 1,000 million. But even there, Jews constitute less than two percent of that population.

Even more remarkable is the number of Jewish-sounding family names one encounters in the arts, in medicine, in biologic science and in physical science and mathematics. Why a disproportionately high fraction of such individuals appear to have Jewish roots is difficult to explain without invoking some genetic basis, but the phenomenon is noticeable even to the casual observer.

Furthermore, the religion itself no longer plays such a large role in the lives of many Jews. I've been an atheist for many years and I think my parents were as well—even though I did undergo ritual circumcision and was Bar-Mitzvah at the usual age of 13. Indeed, the common language in our house when I was a child was Yiddish (because of my grandmother) which I spoke as fluently as English during my pre-teen years.

I should have expected Judaism in the United States to wither away as intermarriage increased and overt persecution and discrimination decreased. Surprisingly there seems to have been a return to Jewish "roots." Why one should continue to profess faith in a God who has allowed Jews to suffer so grievously for so many centuries escapes me. There are of course admirable features of modern (not "orthodox") Judaism—such as its evolution to include women as equal partners, the abiding concern for social justice and equality (which makes it harder for Jews to be Republicans), the emphasis on learning, the recognition that what counts is one's life and deeds here on earth with few illusions about any future "eternal life," the hereafter, heaven and hell, reincarnation, etc. If only the Jews could forget about the "one" God, about Abraham's revelations and God's promises and covenants, and could read the Torah as the human invention it is, rather than being sacred text—but then I suppose they wouldn't be Jews any longer!

Indeed, it would probably be a very good thing if all the monotheistic religions were to disappear and if all the "sacred" texts were unsanctified. There is certainly nothing of value in sacred ("divinely revealed") cosmology, creationism and biology, and little of value in sacred history. All the affirmations about afterlife, heaven, hell, last judgments, etc., are nonsense. The biblical notion that man was created by "God" in His own image and that man is the absolute ruler (by divine right) of all that is in the air, in the seas, and on land is also unjustified. Finally, the injunction to be fruitful and multiply has probably outlived its usefulness.

Science, Medicine, and Religion: For many centuries religion has carried on its wars under the banner of immutable sacred revelation, fighting bitterly and using all possible means to prevent discovery and dissemination of knowledge. Indeed, the tale of Adam and Eve and the Tree of Knowledge seems remarkably revealing. The search for new knowledge is dangerous and costly. The moral is to follow unquestioningly the rules and beliefs passed on from generation to generation as interpreted by priests, imams and other "holy men." Interestingly, the ancient Greeks with their pantheon of gods seem to have been more open-minded and scientifically adventuresome than the monotheists who succeeded them.

The development of heliocentric astronomy removed the planet earth from the center of the universe and further developments have displaced the solar system and mankind to the fringes of the universe. The efforts of physicists and mathematicians to reconcile relativistic gravitation with quantum mechanics in a unified theory is likely to lead to new ways of thinking about cosmology that may no longer require some form of creation such as the "big bang." The recognition of evolution as providing the origin of species, including the recent arrival of *Homo sapiens*, is now underpinned by rapidly increasing understanding of the genetic processes underlying evolution and differentiation of species. ("Creationism" and its many euphemistic synonyms are of course very much alive and well in the United States, and are leading the attack on the teaching of science in the public schools).

The post-double helix biological revolution of the past half-century has profound implications not only for the current and future practice of preventive and therapeutic medicine, but for our understanding of human behavior. The increasing recognition of the importance of genes and of epigenetic mechanisms controlling gene expression as determinants of mental attributes such as personality, intelligence, talent, creativity, etc., will urgently raise serious questions about the axioms upon which we traditionally base the organization of an egalitarian human society.

Furthermore, the tightness of the linkages between male–female coitus, marriage, and the uniqueness of the procreative pathway will need to be rethought. Even the definition of human life will require reconsideration as I attempt to indicate with a few examples below:

211

1. The increasing ability to control human biology with gene therapy or hormonal treatment, or with selection of certain embryos (but not others) destined for full development, allows us to manipulate the characteristics of our children.
2. The cloning of somatic cell nuclei in an enucleated receptor ovum so as to produce embryos and, indeed fully developed organisms, without going through the combination of two haploid gametes undermines our basic notions of procreation. And of course, the use of such artificially created embryonal cell masses as a source of toti-potent embryonal stem cells has aroused much moral fervor and ethical posturing.
3. We have introduced specific human genes into mammalian genomes, and those transgenic hosts express these human genes perfectly well. What about introducing human cell nuclei into enucleated ova of other species?
4. Parthenogenesis is a known phenomenon in "lower" animals, but recently Japanese scientists were able to obtain a few viable mice by the fusion of nuclei from two ova (i.e., no male gamete). This procedure is very complex with a low success rate, so it is not yet ready for prime time, but it is proof of the principle that male gametes are not absolutely required for production of a viable mammal. Two different female gametes can do the job!

Homo sapiens has proven to be an extremely successful species. "Man" has colonized all parts of the planet and multiplied beyond anyone's fondest hopes in only a few thousand generations. And this in spite of epidemic diseases as well as the perpetual carnage associated with human aggression and man's inhumanity to man. This success has been to the detriment of many other species, and we recognize no limits to our right to hunt and kill members of other species. Their evolutionary proximity to man has not protected our closest primate relatives from near-extinction. Nor are other remarkably intelligent mammals such as cetaceans likely to survive.

The Roman Catholic hierarchy continues to make war on all types of birth control or population control other than sexual abstinence, and the Christian Right in the United States seem committed to this war as well. Perhaps the abandonment of our current sacred texts would oblige mankind to reassess its role and its importance relative to other forms of life, and indeed, its responsibilities rather than its privileges.

Monotheistic religions have also contributed to the ethical framework that supports putting a very high value on human life (with many exceptions of course—notably heathens, infidels, apostates, adulterous women, etc.). As physicians we generally do not stint on labor or expense to prolong life and we accept a personal responsibility for each of our patients who has entrusted us with his welfare. The remarkable but costly success of modern medicine in managing many formerly fatal illnesses is raising cost-containment issues at the societal level in prosperous Western societies and is beginning to define the value of human life in monetary and economic units, and to assess the justification for medical treatments on this basis. "Life" itself is no longer the Holy Grail. The "quality" of that life as well as its economic value is increasingly assessed and considered.

I certainly do not have solutions to propose for these many problems. In the long run, unwillingness to assess the realities of scientific discovery and inference on their own merits, rather than through the lens of pre-conceived religious or quasi-religious belief systems, will not help us.

Dr. Bromberg was born in New York City in 1930, the son of immigrants from a southwestern border province of the old Russian empire. He has pursued an academic medical career, directing the divisions of pulmonary/critical care medicine at the Ohio State University College of Medicine and then at the University of North Carolina School of Medicine in Chapel Hill where he also established and directed the Center for Environmental Medicine and Lung Biology. He remains an active faculty member. His principal avocation has been and remains performance of chamber music as a violinist and violist.

Five Essays

A. Scott Earle

On Aging

Happily, we live in a time of lengthening life expectancy. Middle age has been extended, and seventy, eighty and more years are now the norm rather than the exception. Medical advances and good fortune have permitted most of us not only to survive into old age, but also to enjoy our extended lives and even to remain productive. Nevertheless, the platitude that "the best is yet to come" is ridiculous. One pays a price for longevity in the form of degenerative changes affecting both body and mind. Fortunately, innate human adaptability helps us to accept, live with, and work around the humiliating changes that aging brings.

Longevity does confer benefits, even if these are limited. They include increased adaptability, a greater degree of equanimity, elevated pain tolerance, and an experiential honing of judgment (although the latter may be a mixed blessing for, like the curse of Cassandra, it is sometimes difficult to convince others that our judgment indicates better choices).

With increasing age comes increasing awareness that the first shoe has dropped. Waiting for the second one is unproductive and depressing; best to accept, adjust, stay active physically and mentally, and move on as I'll do now, progressing to my next chosen subject.

On Retirement

Retirement did not come easily to me. I agonized about how life would change. By observing others, I could see that there is an ill-defined boundary between middle and old age. People then seem to assume an aura, one that suggests to onlookers that retirement is close at hand. Friends, acquaintances, co-workers, and even complete strangers do not hesitate to ask about retirement plans, a phenomenon that reveals how, when one person drops out, others are affected. Retirement inevitably produces a fault—a gap—in the fabric of society. Who will fill it? And who fills the secondary gap? And so on, like a wave spreading down the occupational pyramid, all the while providing a topic for gossip and speculation.

Retirement affects a retiree in many ways. One accumulates experience, knowledge, judgment, common sense, and just plain know-how during a productive life. These reside in memory; recall requires only an appropriate stimulus. I found it galling to realize that, after a lifetime spent in accumulating these powers, opportunities to use them were nearing an end.

Since reading *The Tempest* while in college, I have been intrigued by the play's premise. It is, to my mind, the best of Shakespeare's plays and it is one to which those who are aging can easily relate. *The Tempest* was the playwright's swan song, written shortly before he left London and the theater for Stratford; he was on the cusp of retirement. Physicians, as they approach retirement, are not unlike Prospero in *The Tempest*. We too have the magic. Hospitals are our islands. Clinics and offices—and, for surgeons, operating rooms—are cells where we exercised our sorcery, where "graves at [our] command have wak'd their sleepers, op'd, and let 'em forth by [our] so potent art." Prospero laments, when the time comes, that "and this rough magic I here abjure . . . I'll break my staff, Bury it certain fathoms in the earth, And deeper than did ever plummet sound I'll drown my book. [*Solemn music*]." (*The Tempest,* V. 1. 48–56)

Power wears different raiments, evidenced by a pleasing deference to the professor and to the older clinician throughout our hospital islands. Renunciation of authority comes with a wrench; a dose of humility is required. Like Prospero, and Shakespeare, one becomes simply an aging citizen. We no longer make sick people well, no longer manage our realms, and no longer impart knowledge. For academics, it means no longer interfacing with students and residents, and no more awed and grateful patients. The line we have walked between life and death suddenly takes on a more personal meaning. We are now "senior citizens," "golden agers," or "honored citizens." Sir George James Frazer was right, when he wrote in *The Golden Bough* that "the king must die." In our time, however, death has been postponed; the king or queen go first to pasture and die later.

Many physicians are able to postpone retirement by "slowing down," an option not open to all. Some are unable to taper off gracefully. In our litigious society, hefty malpractice insurance payments mean that "cutting back" is no longer an option for many—for surgeons especially. Immediate full retirement may be the only choice. Everyone copes in his or her own way. Some become senior statespersons and continue to attend weekly meetings and conferences, maintaining a presence, basking in honors accumulated over the years, tolerated by the impatient young. Others shift into advisory and administrative roles in hospitals, in schools and even in corporate environments. Still others hang it up completely as Shakespeare seems to have done: move to Stratford upon Avon, raise horses, cultivate roses, travel, write books, paint, play golf, construct harpsichords, work with wood, with clay, or just putter; the list of secondary occupations is almost endless. Envy those renaissance persons who are able to switch occupations comfortably. Even if their new lives are not very productive, they bring satisfaction to individuals who are altogether entitled to it.

Belgian anthropologist Arnold van Gennep coined the term "passage rites" in 1909. Since that time ceremonies associated with major change in status have been studied in many societies. Traditionally these are four: birth, coming of age, marriage, and death. All are characterized by anticipation, apprehension, upheaval and change, and all of these exist in the context of retirement. Should not retirement then also be recognized as a true metamorphosis, worthy of appropriate rites? Such might ease the transition from one state to another, and help the retiree recognize his or her emergence into a new world of reduced movie and motel rates, medicare, and more felicitously, a time for writing, for travel and for other cherished pursuits.

I submit that society should now recognize retirement as a *de facto* rite of passage. It should be celebrated with appropriate ceremony, honors, ritual, and panoply. Presently, beyond the occasional award of a watch, we have no established retirement rites—nothing like bar mitzvah, confirmation, public circumcision, tests of bravery, or nuptial ceremony—nothing, in brief, to mark the passage into old age and the pleasures of leisure. I now propose that society should recognize that aging and retirement call for appropriate ceremony. I'm not talking about speeches and engraved watches here. I'm talking about wing-dings, blowouts, and all-out celebration. In short, party time!

On Medicine and Medicines (or: "Ask Your Doctor")

I know about the cost of prescription medicines: my own inter-mittently troublesome allergy along with the aches and pains of osteoarthritis, my spouse's troublesome migraine, horror stories related by relatives and acquaintances about how much they have had to pay for medicines, all add up and have made me acutely aware of how expensive prescription drugs are. I have never been an admirer of the pharmaceutical industry's sale tac-tics—the ads, the office-haunting detail persons bearing gifts of flashlights, pens, key chains, and knick-knacks—but I have lately come to believe that the drug industry is the most grasping and immoral of our nation's businesses. It epitomizes the abuses that can arise within a free-enterprise system, a system that, while encouraging reward, permits excesses detrimental to public wel-fare. The expression, "pigs at a trough," used in a wider context to characterize big business in general, seems especially applica-ble when applied to an industry that seems determined to milk every possible cent from the sale of its products.

Pharmaceutical companies are quick to say that research drives drug prices. Justifiable to a degree, but the high price of prescription drugs goes well beyond that. Ours is the only coun-try that permits advertisements in the popular media—radio, television, newspapers, and magazines—for prescription medica-tions. I have not seen an estimate of how much such advertising costs the lay public, but the figure must be enormous.

Education, both of the medical profession and of the lay public, could do much to lower costs. Physicians should be made fully aware that many heavily promoted drugs are molec-ularly closely related to older ones, and in some cases offer no advantage to patients over parent formulations. The delayed action proton-pump inhibitor Nexium (esomeprazole magne-sium), one of many effective medications for the treatment of gastro-esophageal reflux disease, is an outstanding example. Television and magazines in the recent past have been flooded with impressive "ask your doctor" ads for the "purple pill." Aggressive advertising has added greatly to its cost. If medical organizations actively discouraged doctors from prescribing Nex-ium and other heavily advertised drugs, and if insurers and groups such as the AARP discouraged patients from requesting them, the pharmaceutical industry might get the message and modify their advertising practices.

While getting a drug to market is undeniably expensive, the initial research, which the industry claims is one reason for high drug prices, is often initiated and carried out in university or government laboratories. Procrit (erythropoietin) is an example. It is an injectable medication used to treat anemia; it costs approximately $500 for each injection. Procrit has been heavily advertised both on television and in popular magazines as a "call your doctor" drug for patients undergoing chemotherapy. Surely the decision to use such a potent and expensive medication is one that should be left to the treating oncologist, rather than by patient-directed advertisements. (Ironically, it has recently been suggested that erythropoietin may adversely affect the action of chemotherapeutic agents!)

Physicians, from whom all prescriptions emanate, could also help to lower the cost of medications by the simple expedient of selective prescription. As physicians know—although many do not act on the knowledge—some older generic drugs are equal to, and sometimes even more effective than newer, far more expensive ones. In the treatment of allergy (a condition in which I am obviously interested), the heavily advertised Claritin (loratidine) is much more expensive, and less effective (for some patients, ineffective), than are older medications such as Chlortrimeton (chlorpheniramine) and Benadryl (diphenhydramine). Certainly these generic compounds should be tried before writing a prescription for a heavily advertised and less effective second-generation antihistamine. Chlortrimeton's side effects, have—for obvious reasons—been stressed in lay advertisements by the makers of Claritin, Zyrtec (cetirizine) and Allegra (fexofenadine), yet there is no convincing evidence that they are any greater than are those of the second-generation medications; indeed, effectiveness and mild sedation may be inseparable. Similarly, Diuril (chlororthiazide) and its congeners, drugs that have been around since the 1950s, are usually a better choice for treating patients with mild hypertension than are newer, far more expensive ones. Physicians should be encouraged to look hard and critically at all drugs that are advertised directly to the public before prescribing them. Is it unreasonable to consider patients' pocketbooks as well as their presenting conditions?

Medical organizations and their members also owe it to the public to lobby against drug advertising directed at consumers, rather than at the medical profession. We should fight legislative measures that blatantly favor drug manufacturers at patient expense. Politicians accept large donations from the pharmaceutical industry, but is that a reason to pass legislation that prevents governmental agencies from negotiating drug costs, as the Bush administration has done with the recently passed Prescription Drug Act? (It is not surprising to learn that the head of the FDA until recently was George W. Bush's campaign manager's brother—and that the agency aggressively sought to curtail purchase of drugs from Canada.) Finally, we all should unite to help to remove an administration that permits and seemingly encourages an out-of-control pharmaceutical industry to exploit our citizens.

Addendum: After writing the above, I learned that the AARP (an organization from which I resigned in disgust over their support of the Prescription Drug Act) pledged to act on all of the points mentioned in the preceding essay (*AARP Bulletin,* 8:42, February 2004). I have rejoined.

The Bush Administration: A Short Quiz

There is no way of escaping the impact that the Iraq war—now over, but not finished—has had on our country. In trying to write about it, I find that outrage and anger have tempered every word that pops up on my computer screen. I can't guess how widely what we have written here will be read, but I take this opportunity to let posterity know that there *are* Americans who are fully aware of the Bush administration's immorality. In watching what it has done to our country and the world, I have come to believe that many Germans must have had the same feeling of helplessness during Hitler's ascendancy. Happily, we Americans have the power to depose bad leaders.

In the spring of 2003 the United States invaded a sovereign nation, one that did not represent a threat to our country or the world. It was, it seems, a long contemplated invasion based on arrogance, and faulty, selectively applied intelligence. In so doing, the United States alienated the United Nations and the people and governments of the world. With his "preemptive war" George W. Bush made the most grievous and unjustifiable mistake in the history of the American presidency.

I lie awake thinking of questions that I would like ask George W. Bush and those who support him:

Q: Isn't an invasion by any name still an invasion? Is the invasion of Iraq any less an invasion than, say, Hitler's invasion of Poland? (As Ms. Stein might have said; "an invasion is an invasion is an invasion. . . . ")

Q: Answer honestly, now: wasn't the war expected to stimulate a slow economy by tooling up war industries, and by supporting airlines, faltering after 9/11? Hundreds of thousands of men, women, and their equipment flying to and from Iraq really gave the airlines a boost. It also gave the term "mass transportation" a new and very expensive meaning!

Q: Do George W. Bush and those around him care that the world sees their war in Iraq as an attempt to control the world's largest deposit of oil? Is our country really in a position to ignore world opinion so blithely?

Q: If America had been invaded wouldn't we characterize Americans who opposed the foreign invader as "freedom fighters"? Why do we characterize Iraqis who fight a foreign invader as "terrorists"? (Interestingly, many who protested the war predicted that guerilla warfare would erupt as the war ended.)

Q: By what miracle of rationalization can an avowed bornagain Christian live with the knowledge that he has unjustifiably caused the deaths of thousands?

Q: What of the wounded and maimed? Not much has been said about them. How can George W. Bush and his administration legitimize their immediate agony and permanent crippling in the face of the revelation that there were no weapons of mass destruction, that Iraq did not represent an imminent threat to us or its neighbors, and that there was no connection between Iraq and the terrorists of 9/11?

Q: Do those who brought us this war ever consider the immense waste of the world's resources and America's wealth? Imagine what could have been done with those resources had they been used to better our country's infrastructure, to educate our children, to improve a failing environment, and to export American aid peacefully to others?

Q. Finally, does George W. Bush realize he is now part of a prevalent list of anathematic terms; terms like "body parts," "suicide bombers," "body count," "weapons of mass destruction," "nuclear fallout," "dirty bomb," "terminal care," and now "Bush administration"?

As I re-read the above, I see that what I wrote is truly invective. Nevertheless it gives outlet to my anger. Words can go only so far in describing my contempt for George W. Bush and those in government who have encouraged and supported his actions. There is some comfort in knowing that there is at least a possibility that he will be deprived of another term. By the time this appears in print, I will know; in the meantime I will pray.

Addendum: The above, written prior to the last presidential election, described my disgust for a callous, dishonest administration—in the interim it has only worsened. If a people deserves the leaders that it gets, what does this imply about those who made George W. Bush's re-election possible?

The Environment

While studying bacteriology, I asked one of our Nobel laureate teachers what happened to bacteria left to themselves, undisturbed, to multiply in a Petri dish. One of two things, he said: either they die, killed by the poison of their own metabolites, or they exist indefinitely without multiplying in deviant and mutated form (although, encouragingly, they retain the ability to return to a healthy state when conditions warrant).

Following completion of my surgical residency, I moved to Idaho and practiced there from the late 1950s into the 1970s. We still spend our summers there, in the conjoined Ketchum/Sun Valley area. The community lies at an altitude of six thousand feet (mid-elevation in this mountainous state), and is located in the central part of Idaho, eighty miles north of the Snake River. Even after I gave up my practice in Idaho in the early 1970s for further training in plastic and reconstructive surgery, we returned every year on vacation. Now, since I have retired, we spend half of each year there. One of the advantages of aging is that it permits us to see trends over time that are lost on others. Here are some observations based on a lengthy residence in a mountain community.

Last summer, as we do every year, we followed a rough, four-wheel drive road high up into the Pioneer Range in Central Idaho. We parked our Pathfinder, and set out on foot. The trail led us to a pass that topped 9000 feet where we were rewarded with a magnificent view of sheer cliffs, waterfalls, and hanging valleys of the Pioneers. We scrambled even higher, up a steep talus slope above tree line. Here, to our surprise, we encountered tall wide-leaved, conically shaped plants with terminal spikes bearing clustered flowers. They were green gentians or monument plants, *Frasera speciosa,* a plant common on valley floors and side slopes. Now, here they were, higher up than we had ever seen them before, in a location that was in former years colder and less conducive to growth. The plants are, in effect, migrating northward.

Much else has changed in our mountains during the past fifty years. In the 1960s, we expected snow every month of the year—it never snows now in the summer. Snowfields used to persist year-round as mini-glaciers—no more, for the summer's heat melts the snow by the first of August. Daytime summer temperatures in the valleys seldom used to reach 90°F. Recently, however, temperatures have stayed at 100° day after day during summer months. We formerly slept under blankets all year-round and it would have been too cold to climb high while wearing only short-sleeved shirts and shorts as we do today. We would have been reluctant then to climb above treeline without carrying gloves, parka, and a sweater in our packs.

These observations, I agree, are anecdotal. Nevertheless, given the time span over which we have been there, they seem to mirror the climatic changes that are affecting the world. Their validity is supported by the scientific confirmation of global warming. Many still deny that the world's atmosphere is changing; or if it is, they believe that the changes are benign. Doubters are able to martial plenty of evidence against climate change, derived from short-term observations. However persuasive these may seem, there is now unequivocal evidence of a long-term warming trend, one that has been more rapid in recent years. (See Spencer R. Weart, *The Discovery of Global Warming,* Harvard University Press, 2003: a dispassionate, well-documented, historical account of research leading up to the recognition of world climate change.) Here are some other indications, based on changes that have occurred in our lifetime:

Item: Seventy-five years ago there were over one hundred glaciers in Montana's Glacier National Park; there are 35 today. At the present rate of recession these will all be gone in three or four decades.

Item: Mount Kilimanjaro's much-publicized snowcap is disappearing. If it continues to melt at the present rate the snowcap will disappear completely in fifteen years.

Item: Glacial retreat is pronounced in Alaska. Some glaciers have retreated as much as seven miles in recent times. Andean glaciers are also disappearing rapidly. Similarly, the arctic icepack is thinning and breaking up earlier each year. It has been predicted, if melting continues at its present rate, that the North Pole will soon lie in open water.

Item: frozen tundra ("permafrost") in the Arctic is melting and being colonized by shrubs. Plant and animal ranges are moving slowly northward each year (and southward, too, in the antipodes).

Item: the number of penguins that nest on Antarctic ice is showing a decrease; the opposite is true for open water species that nest on dry ground. Similarly, populations of migratory birds dependent on seasonal temperature regularity are threatened: scientists predict extinctions. And the list could go on.

The specter of increasing global temperature is disturbing, as uncertainty always is. The uncertainty is not *whether* the climate is changing; the uncertainty relates to what changes global warming will bring. There is no way to make accurate predictions, for there is no way of knowing how the climate will react to continued, uncontrolled atmospheric pollution and conversion of fossil fuels into carbon dioxide. The only certainty is change itself. Rapid climate swings, sometimes over a very short time, are known to have occurred in the past; there is even some small chance, apparently, that the earth might experience compensatory cooling.

There is no question about what needs to be done: foremost we should curtail the use of fossil fuel, and work to remove particulate material from the atmosphere. (See James Hansen, Defusing the Global Warming Time Bomb, *Scientific American*, 290: no. 3: 68–77.) Nuclear power might help over a short term, but sources of renewable energy are needed: wind, solar energy, ocean tides, geothermal are all possibilities. Unfortunately, these are only band-aiding, for uncontrolled population growth is of course the ultimate cause of climate change. When we were born, three quarters of a century ago, only a few neo-Malthusians saw population growth as an evil. Nuclear war, environmental degradation, global warming were unrecognized threats then. So much has changed!

~

Now, I am standing on a mountain that looks down on the community where I lived, and practiced. It was little more than a village in the 1950s, with a permanent population of only seven hundred people (in nearby communities, others farmed, raised cattle and sheep, mined, and lumbered: these were our patients). If one includes seasonal variations, the population of the Ketchum/Sun Valley area has increased almost ten-fold during the ensuing years; the figure would be higher had developers been able to find more room for building in the narrow valley.

From where I am standing I can see the north–south main highway, State Route 75. To the north lies the Sawtooth National Recreation Area, a spectacular mountainous region with montane and subalpine forests, chains of alpine lakes, and the Salmon River Valley. A discrete haze of pollution snakes along the road above an endless stream of the cars, trucks, and campers. With the arrival of summer, roadside campgrounds fill with campers and trailers. Trailhead parking lots are filled with cars from dozens of states. The most scenic spots in the high mountains are now dotted with bright backpacker's tents during much of the summer.

Literally hundreds of plant species bloom in Idaho's mountains, including spectacular blue gentians, Lewis' mountain flax, yellow monkey-flowers, colorful wild buckwheat, and clumps of lily-like white mountain camas. Unfortunately these are too often flattened by hikers' boots. Almost every hanging valley has one or more lovely mountain lakes, although some are now forming algal blooms because the water is "enriched" by human and animal waste. ATVs (all-terrain vehicles) cruise many of the trails leading to the high country, fouling the air with their exhaust (ATVs and snowmobiles burn a noxious oil-gasoline mixture).

The effects of heavy use are clear, widespread, and disheartening. They are seen everywhere in the West. Yellowstone Park in Wyoming, Montana's Glacier National Park, Yosemite in California,

Utah's Bryce and Zion parks are now so crowded with visitors that controlled visitation is in place. Winter pollution by snowmobiles in Yellowstone Park is so severe that park personnel at entry points wear masks, while others try to keep the snowmobilers from chasing down snowbound elk, deer and buffalo. The impact of crowding on our recreational lands, of developments in wild places, and of increasing degradation of rivers is the result of the population growth that has occurred, mostly since the end of World War II.

Obviously, the twin evils of worldwide environmental degradation and global warming must be controlled if our descendants are to have decent lives. And it is the earth's human population that drives both. Consider that the world's population has increased from three to six billion since 1960 and that three billion more are predicted by 2050. Ignorance, coupled with peculiar faith-based religious convictions in America and elsewhere, make it unlikely that population growth will be controlled in the foreseeable future. Tragically, catastrophic determinants are standing in the wings waiting to do the job. Animal disease is spreading to humans; Nile virus has spread to the United States from Africa as has AIDS. The latter has caused millions of deaths there, with millions more expected. There is nothing to prevent tropical diseases—malaria, dengue fever and others—from becoming endemic in yesterday's temperate zones. Influenza spreads from animals to humans in Asia and then throughout the world; crowding encourages spread. A recurrence of the 1918 influenza pandemic is the most frightening scenario of all, and the chances of a similar disaster in the future are very real.

In the past, Black Death (bubonic plague), cholera and consumption (tuberculosis) effectively reduced populations in crowded cities. Now, much of the world is crowded and will become more so. Smallpox, purposely seeded, or from spontaneous genetic modification of animal?? pox could spread through the world's population leaving death, blindness and scarring in its wake. Entire native populations were wiped out after the disease was introduced into the New World from Europe. Cortez, Pizarro and North American settlers had a powerful ally in smallpox. Natural disasters are also having dire effects in heavily populated areas. As an example, I spent several months in Armenia in the early 1990s, establishing a plastic surgical center in the capital, Yerevan. Its primary purpose was to aid mutilated survivors of the Armenian earthquake of December 1988, in which between fifty and one hundred thousand people died. (Unsettled political events at the time prevented more accurate casualty figures.)

Reason suggests that it would be more merciful to control human population by planning, rather than for our descendants to go the way of bacteria in a closed Petri dish. It is vital that all nations recognize and accept the challenges posed by a deteriorating environment and a burgeoning population. Regrettably, the Bush administration has refused to recognize that environmental changes and uncontrolled population growth are a threat to coming generations. The United States, both as the world's wealthiest country, and by far its biggest polluter, should be leading the fight against further environmental degradation. Unfortunately these responsibilities have been dodged. George W. Bush's refusal either to sign the Kyoto Treaty, or to offer a reasonable alternative, is deplorable and dangerous.

On the bright side, humans are adaptive and we do tend to muddle through. The world may have to wait until deleterious effects of a changing environment become obvious, but, when these are finally recognized, people will act. We can only hope that the call to action comes before the oceans start to boil, and that our descendants praise rather than curse those who preceded them on planet Earth.

Addendum: Since writing this essay about the environment two years ago, natural disasters, a tsunami, hurricanes, and earthquakes have struck populous areas around the globe, with devastating loss of human life. As population and crowding increase we should expect even greater mortality as a sequela of natural disaster. The same may be expected with global diseases; as I write this SARS has missed, and H5N1 influenza is in a holding pattern. And the world's population has continued to increase. . . .

Dr. Earle's love of mountains developed in Colorado while serving in the Army's 10th Mountain Division during World War II. He later trained in surgery at the Peter Bent Brigham Hospital. After ten years of surgical practice in Idaho he trained further in plastic surgery atCleveland's University Hospitals. He retired as Professor of (Plastic) Surgery from Case Western Reserve School of Medicine. Since, he has authored books on Idaho's mountain flora and (with James L. Reveal, Ph.D.) on the plants of the Lewis and Clark expedition.

Through the Retrospectoscope and Beyond

Edwin W. Brown

The opening line of an old hymn, sung in the church of my childhood—"From Greenland's icy mountains to India's coral strands"—presaged the inception of a career that was to expose me to a world of which I was abysmally ignorant, save for a stint in the military in Italy during World War II. Two summers in a village in northern Greenland while a student at the Harvard School of Public Health was soon followed by two years of teaching preventive medicine in India, the latter resulting in an interest in medical education in developing countries that defined the remainder of my medical career.

The peripatetic wanderings of a professional traveler brings one in touch with the gamut of humankind, from presidents, kings, and even the last of the world's emperors in their mansions or palaces to the most humble peasant in his hut of mud and straw—with the realization that there is not much difference among them. They live and they die, and what each leaves behind is often not all that perceptible whatever their station in life.

If I have learned anything from traveling the world, it is the inescapable frailty of life, and in particular, for those in high position. Not long after my having met His Imperial Majesty Mohammad Reza Pahlavi in his palace in Tehran, this Shahanshah (King of Kings) became a wandering exile with terminal cancer. Similarly, as director of a humanitarian aid project in Vietnam, I met Lyndon Johnson in the Oval Office early in the war that eventually ended his political career and left him a broken man. (Lest I might have been seen as the personification of *Li'l Abner's* Joe Btfsplk, I refrain from commenting at length on one of my visits to Afghanistan in which King Zahir Shah was overthrown four hours after my departure, or leaving Baghdad the day its erstwhile president was scheduled for assassination.)

229

As physicians, we are, of course, only too well aware of how quickly a promising life can be snuffed out by accident or disease. Yet how many of us have been outspoken in our condemnation of abortion on demand, a practice that has ended the lives of millions of healthy human beings in this country in recent decades, and that by our fellow physicians? Thus far we have largely avoided the travesty now legalized in the Netherlands that is responsible for ending life at the other end of the age spectrum, again by our fellow physicians, but recent legislation in Oregon suggests we may be heading in that direction.

On the positive side, life in the latter half of the twentieth century was an exciting adventure. We put men on the moon, and through deep space probed the unimaginably vast expanse of the universe. Advances in medicine have exceeded the wildest dreams of those who preceded us in the first half of the century. Although life for many Americans in recent years has been financially trying, even the poorest of us enjoy a standard of living that exceeds by far that of vast numbers of our fellow humans in many other countries.

But where are we headed? In the midst of all our prosperity our society is rapidly undergoing profound changes that are undermining much of the good we've been able to accomplish in health care, racial equality, social reform, and virtually any other area of life one might mention. In just a few short years we have seen startling examples of corporate corruption at the highest levels, unprecedented outbursts of deadly anger among our youth, and alcohol and drug abuse extending from areas of urban squalor into our most privileged suburbs and remotest communities. Qualitatively, none of this is new, but the quantitative aspects are frightening. Some would take the media to task for constantly parading all this before us and thus encouraging more of the same deviant behavior among those so inclined. Others would have us believe that things are not really as bad as they seem; what has always been is simply being brought to light through vastly improved methods of communication.

As this is being written, our Supreme Court is being asked to decide whether the words "under God" should remain in our Pledge of Allegiance; yet to a man, those who drafted the Declaration of Independence and the Constitution affirmed their belief in God and the absolute necessity of divine law as the governing force in the life of the country and its citizens. Moreover, as Senator Bill Frist, a distinguished member of our profession, pointed out in defense of a constitutional amendment forbidding same-sex marriage, the only reason the constitution makes no mention of such is that our forefathers never dreamed that such an issue could ever arise.

Indeed, how many of us could ever have dreamed even a decade or so ago that junior high school girls in some of our communities have taken on a new challenge seeing who can perform the most acts of oral sex on boys while on the school bus? Or that in many of our primary schools the conventional wisdom of many of our educators is that children just out of kindergarten need to be taught the dangers of anal sex?

And what has happened to those absolutes of morality instilled in us by our parents—the Judeo–Christian principles on which this country was founded? Even among some of the most conservative religious groups in our country, teenagers today believe everything to be relative. "If it feels good and does no harm to others, it's okay!" The problem is, of course, that they have no concept of what harm it can do to others.

To avoid expanding the litany of complaints with which all of us are only too familiar, let me turn to an examination of what I see as hopeful in all of this. One of the most profound events in our lifetime has been the rise and fall of an evil that not many years ago was rapidly taking over much of the world. Today, while the largest nation in the world still retains a Communist government, its leaders have recognized the utter failure of Marxist economic policies, resulting in a surge of capitalism second to none. The expansion of industry and business in China is nothing short of phenomenal. "Made in China" appears on even the most sophisticated technological equipment we import, retail sales outlets there are multiplying at an incredible rate (there's even a Starbucks in the Forbidden City in Beijing), and China is developing a huge middle class. During a February 2004 visit, my wife and I saw almost no foreigners in Beijing, Kunming, Xian, and Tianjin, nor on any of the flights taken between those cities, yet every MacDonald, KFC, or Pizza Hut we passed (and there are hundreds of them in Beijing alone) were filled with Chinese.

Far more important, however, is what we learned about religious life in China. The spiritual bankruptcy of Communism has resulted in massive conversions to Christianity in recent years—by Beijing government estimates at a rate of more than 30,000 a day, despite continuing harassment by hard-line local officials, imprisonment of leaders of the unregistered house churches (now with a total following of an estimated 60 million), and well-documented cases of torture of some thus imprisoned. Even among the registered Protestant and Catholic churches, which enjoy remarkable freedom in their worship services despite government controls, the membership has increased to more than 30 million.

Moreover, this phenomenal growth is entirely "home-grown." Missionaries are not allowed into China, nor are the Chinese churches permitted to have close ties with any foreign religious body, although the Catholics are allowed to identify themselves with the Papacy in Rome. The registered Protestant churches belong to the Three Self Patriotic Movement—self-supporting, self-governing, self-propagating.

Chinese intellectuals played a major role in shaping the nation's destiny in the twentieth century, from the overthrow of the Ch'ing Dynasty in 1911 to and since the Tiananmen Square massacre in 1989, and many academics are embracing Christianity in their search for truth and justice. Truth, as an absolute, is largely lacking in the Chinese philosophies of Buddhism, Taoism, or Confucianism, and these intellectuals have found a lack of sound ideology in Marxism.

An estimated twenty percent of the world's population lives in China, and China enjoys the fastest-growing economy in the world today. In the late '90s the Chinese Academy of Sciences was reported as having predicted that the fastest growing religion in China in the new millennium would be Christianity, a prediction rapidly being fulfilled—and added that this was good, because "a good Christian is a good Chinese." If this growth continues at the present rate, the majority of Chinese will be Christians in the next twenty years. If such should prove to be the case, its implications for the world as a whole are enormous.

Whatever the past perversions of the teachings of Christ by the organized church, and there have been many, the spread of that religion through the most undeveloped countries of the world brought with it medical care and other humanitarian aid that set the standard for what eventually followed under self-government. Even today, the Christian hospitals in many of those countries are among the finest. But the growth of the church in these countries has had a far more profound effect on the lives of many of its citizens than improvement in their health facilities. Uganda, for example, one of the hardest hit by AIDS in Africa, has experienced a dramatic turnaround in its AIDS problem through the efforts of its president in enlisting the support of church leaders in promoting abstinence among the youth, together with marital fidelity and other family values.

What does this have to do with China? The sixty million or so members of the house churches are unanimous in their commitment to send vast numbers of their younger people into the Muslim, Hindu, and Buddhist countries to the west of China to settle in communities throughout these countries, ministering to the needs of the underprivileged and fully prepared to die if their humanitarian efforts are rejected by the militant factions in other religions. Having been brought into the Christian faith as the result of the efforts of missionaries of old, many of whom were martyred, they feel an intense obligation to share what they have been privileged to receive from the God whom they worship. The impact of such commitment could have a most profound effect on that troubled area of the world.

Our founding fathers were unequivocal in their commitment to Judeo–Christian principles as the foundation of our government and our society. Yet while the vast majority of Americans affirm belief in God, and most claim commitment to these Judeo–Christian principles, there is a pervasive atmosphere of condemnation of religious expression within our society. As Senate Majority Leader Frist said in a recent interview, "We are a pluralist nation, as we should be. Government can't make people religious or devout, but it can and must get out of the way and let religion flourish. Attempts to denude the public square of all religious expression betray a misunderstanding of the role of religion in a pluralist nation." "Diversity" is the watchword of the politically correct who loudly demand "tolerance" yet they are manifestly intolerant of those who would share publicly the faith that could immeasurably improve the lives of others as it has theirs.

The ancient book of Job describes a cosmic struggle between the God of creation and the fallen angel, Lucifer, who sought to become as God. Many millennia later that cosmic struggle manifests itself in the determination of a militant group within a major world religion who would destroy all that America represents and are not averse to destroying the innocent among their own people in the process. May we as a nation give no ground in opposing this evil, confident that the God who created us and them is still in control. Placing our hope in any other than that same God is futile. As Abraham Lincoln said to one who asked if God was on his side, "Sir, my concern is not whether God is on our side. My great concern is to be on God's side."

After receiving a Master of Public Health degree and completing the course for teachers of preventive medicine at the Harvard School of Public Health, Dr. Brown spent three years in the Department of Preventive Medicine of Tufts University School of Medicine, followed by two years as visiting professor of preventive medicine at Osmania University, Hyderabad, India. The remainder of his career was devoted to assisting in the development of medical schools in the Middle East and South Asia.

Feminine Reflections

Iolanda Einstein Low

There are two characteristics of individuals that are difficult to hide: skin color and sex. They have a dramatic effect on one's life. As a white woman I can only attest to the significant effects of possessing the XX chromosome in the twentieth century. Some of the experiences were wonderful, but unfortunately too many were painful and unjust. Fortunately many situations are changing but not rapidly enough, especially for the millions of women across the world whose aspirations are only impossible dreams. The role of females and the relationship between males and females in our world has been the subject of historical inquiries, speculation, and prejudice since time immemorial. The perceptions of the female role delineated mostly by the more dominant males in most societies and especially in religions have been varied, often contradictory, and still today under heated discussion and prejudice. Few have been more heated than the role of women in medicine.

Personal Reflections after Fifty Years

The seven women who were part of the 110 students admitted to Harvard Medical School's (HMS) class of 1953 (our ranks grew to a total of 140 students on graduation) were extremely visible and under scrutiny. As this was only the fifth class that had been admitted since 1945, many were concerned that this post-WWII decision was wrong. I will never forget the first words I heard on my way to registration: "God damn you for coming here! Women don't belong at HMS. If the 'good men' had not gone to war, the Faculty would have never allowed the 'others' to give in to the pressure of admitting women."

Even after overcoming the hurdles before, during, and after medical school, women were kept under a microscope. We were

235

watched to see whether we were truly competent and caring doctors and thus had not usurped the places traditionally filled by males. Though much has changed, HMS reunion reports show that doubts and questions linger. On the twenty-fifth anniversary of the admission of women to HMS, the report "Worthy of the Honor" still questioned whether "HMS had done the right thing" without the possible neglect and damage to the traditional role of women regarding marriage, child bearing, and family responsibilities.

Despite the increasing presence of women in medicine, the fiftieth reunion report for the class of 1953 queried as to whether women changed medicine or whether women, having been involved in the process of medical training, have changed, perhaps being molded to fit into the standard role. Not all classmates responded, though many had been unaware that their female classmates had any adverse experiences until their daughters or other relatives aspired to become physicians. A few still worried about the conflict with family responsibilities, but most felt the women had a positive affect on the practice of medicine without having to change their personalities. My response to the question posed in 2003 was:

> "Today, in part due to the presence of women in medicine, there is a greater concern for the patient as a human being rather than a diagnosis; there is also concern for the needs of the deliverers of medical care whether student or physician, to assure his or her well being, mentally and physically, with fewer hours on call, support services, more liberal options for part-time work, family, etc. Of course when we graduated, the few women were expected to follow the long-standing pattern as defined by the male gender. . . ."[1]

Also their professional choices upon graduation were often limited to pediatrics and psychiatry, considered the more "caring" professions. Fortunately we've benefited from the societal changes during the feminine movement in the 1960s resulting in the passage of the 1972 Federal Act addressing inequalities in the work place. Thus the disappearance of the "separate but equal rule" resulted in a significant breakthrough for women and minorities. Today, in medicine, gender seems not to be an issue except for the glass ceiling in academia in the United States.

Reflections on History

Because the past continues to influence our perceptions of women today in many societies, I have been fascinated in examining the constant contradiction of the portrayal of women and their aspirations throughout history. It is important to remember that history, including many religious views, has been written mostly by men!

Our Judeo–Christian heritage, as represented by the Bible, describes many fascinating but often not very admirable women. In the Old Testament there is Eve, a combination of sexuality, ambition, selfishness, and occasional greed, presenting, with others, a very negative picture of women. In contrast to Eve, the New Testament presents Mary, the Madonna, as the ideal mother figure, both humble and saintly, for over 2000 years. But in general the New Testament has little encouraging to say about women. They should be silent, listen, and learn quietly and submissively; as "men are the leaders."

The Greco Roman period admired Penelope, the faithful wife, awaiting the return of an unfaithful Odysseus. Another mother figure was the Roman matriarch, Cornelia of the Gracchis, who when asked why she wore no jewels proudly presented her two children as her jewels. She needed no other adornment. A less motherly, but better known figure at the time of Rome was the seductive Cleopatra, queen of Egypt, who did play an important historical role.

In China, the concept of Yin and Yang defined the female aspect as weaker, somewhat darker, and softer side than the contrasting male half. From the Middle Ages when a woman's lot was as chattel or as servant, without much power, there emerges, however, an ethereal Beatrice who in the *Divina Comedia* was the beautiful guide who lets Dante reach paradise. Then there is also the saintly but far more war-like Joan of Arc who sacrifices her life for god-like visions and patriotism.

By the sixteenth century a striking contrast to the contemporary role of women was the strong, powerful but certainly not saintly monarch Elizabeth I of England who defended Britain and the future of its sea power. It is interesting that in Shakespeare's plays of that era the roles of women, though played by men, were portrayed as stronger, more admirable persons. Less admirable were the women during the French Revolution who sat at the guillotine watching avidly as heads rolled into baskets.

The nineteenth century witnessed the powerful impact of another female ruler in Britain and its empire. Victoria Regina, wife and mother, had fixed ideas of morality, women's role, family life, and dress code that had an immense effect on women. She probably would have dismissed the excesses of the French revolution as an aberration of too much freedom expounded by the French philosophy of *egalité* and not worthy of English womanhood.

Back to Medicine

Despite the restraints of the Victorian Era, there were a number of writers, artists, and political activists battling for the vote, financial independence, and professional recognition. Among them were courageous women who braved ridicule, overt hostility and continual rejections from the mid-1800s in order to obtain an MD degree. This obstinate "male aggressive" behavior of women on both sides of the Atlantic slowly changed the admission policies of many medical schools by first allowing women to attend courses despite vigorous objections from many professors, and eventually allowing full matriculation.

By 1895, even Vienna, then one of the foremost centers of medicine, was drawn into the heated debate on the acceptability of admitting women into the rigorous study of medicine. My research into that period of controversy was prompted by the fact that another Dr. Low (my father-in-law) was a male student at that time. In addition many of the arguments regarding the status of women bore a striking resemblance to discussions fifty years later at HMS. The horrified opposition cautioned that it would destroy the quality and morality of the profession, and, at the same time offend the natural modesty of true womanhood whose natural destiny was to become wife, mother, and protector of the home. The comments that female applicants were mannish, sexually repressed, frustrated, and not fit to be in normal society seem comical today. Those few who succeeded in becoming physicians were pointed out as "the exceptions that proved the rule."

The indignation was sufficient for a surgeon to publish a collection of observations on the female species, which he considered to be psychologically and physically different with a smaller brain thus lacking the intellectual depths and the logical and emotional stability of a man. Thus the study of medicine for women was an absurdity. To quote from his monograph: "Everything of worth in human life that you see around you has been the work of men from the time you get up in the morning and use throughout the day and evening for your comfort. It is the order of society: all is the work of men!"[2] Another quote: "I will say, since the time of Eve in paradise, in the whole world during thousand of years despite millions of women not one ever had a serious thought or action in contrast to what men had thought or achieved."[3]

Dr. Albert, the surgeon, continued to describe the horrors that would befall his daughter if she had to study with males in the demanding medical courses. This would include examining naked bodies, dissecting corpses, taking care of the "lower orders," while trying to keep up, physically and morally, without damaging her ability to remain a "true" female accepted in society.

This negative view of women was not helped by the analyses of many women by Dr. Sigmund Freud on his famous couch in Vienna. From his studies he felt they were superficial, hysterical beings. The uterus was targeted as the causative organ of female depression and "over heated," illogical emotions. The suggestion that penis envy early in infancy caused many of the psychological ills of the "weaker sex" has itself caused continuing controversy.

Despite the vigorous opposition, the University of Vienna admitted women for the full four-year course, graduating their first MDs in 1900. While other medical institutions also admitted women, HMS remained a bastion of ultra-conservatism for another fifty years. The school's arguments remained steadfast from the 1800s that women would destroy their school as well as the profession by their presence alone. How could the men of Harvard allow their wives and daughters to tarnish their family life, their sensitive natures? How could they possibly undertake the rigor of patient care with their limited understanding, knowledge, and delicate anatomy? Nursing and midwifery could be allowed for some members of the "lower classes" under the direction of properly accredited male physicians.

From time to time, feelings escalated into full-scale demonstrations against the "amalgamation of sexes and races." In 1853 the establishment of the New England Female Medical College caused some consternation, especially among obstetricians, as a serious inroad by female professionals. Somewhat later, an offer of $10,000 in 1878 was eventually rejected as being too risky with the recommendation to use the funds for an independent women's medical college that eventually could be brought into the university as a separate college. This was never implemented but the "separate but equal" conditions survived at the university in many forms until a federal law for equality in the workplace was passed in 1972. It should be noted that Johns Hopkins accepted a different grant of money that stipulated the admission of women to its medical school because of serious financial need at the end of the 19th century! Then World War I provided the first wedge into HMS male conservatism with a proposal to admit women due to the war-time shortage of appropriate male candidates. With the war ending, the proposal died. However the post-war era had brought significant changes in society including the economical and political status of women. Those pioneer women MDs in the 1920s and 1930s, whose ability and dedication were not questioned, were still considered unfeminine as many remained unmarried or limited their family responsibilities to a single child. At Harvard, faculty records continued to show the same negative phrases that had been already heard in the University of Vienna's debates in 1894. Thus the consensus that HMS should remain "free of women" was continued until the mid 1940s.

World War II brought back the need for qualified applicants. No longer was it questioned whether women were too weak physically, faint hearted, or not intelligent enough to help in the war effort, but even in 1943 the faculty vote continued to be unfavorable. Finally, in 1944 it was decided that it was preferable to admit qualified women rather then unqualified men.

Reflections on the Present and Future

Finally, in 1945, twelve "superbly qualified women" were admitted to HMS. These past fifty years have seen welcome changes in medicine from the few to fifty percent of admissions, no longer in a separate category, accepted in academia, with an improving wage structure, accommodation to child bearing and rearing, and accessibility to all specialties. This had not been true for the early graduates who chose the most welcoming fields of pediatrics and psychiatry.

Unfortunately there were "by-products" from the changes in women's roles. As "women's lib" became fashionable, it was used as an excuse for undesirable attributes or roles for women: sexual exploitation, unhealthy lifestyles resulting in increased incidence of sexually transmitted diseases and drug use, as well as glorification of the selfish and "materialistic" individualism. Such destructive masochistic forces underline the need to guard what has been gained. The current generations of women in medicine have only a vague notion, often a disbelief, of the obstacles that women had to overcome to become physicians. For those who say, "it can't happen here" they should look at other countries in today's world where a woman can lose her legal status, financial rights as well as being confined in her home and ruled by her husband. Such normal activities for the western women as driving a car, traveling within her country, choosing her education, profession and even the ability to have normal contact with other men would be severely restricted if not punished. Everyday we see women whose faces and bodies are enveloped in ugly and awkward garments that not only hide their femininity but also turn them into non-persons, possessions of men often less valued then animals.

Conclusions

After reflecting on the many views and facets of women over the ages, the question remains for many: "who am I?" My answer today would be that perhaps I am a complex mosaic with some qualities not much different from my male colleagues. Thus I remain intellectually driven, curious about life, thirsting for knowledge, striving to succeed, and above all, wanting "to do good." My feminine side, on the other hand, has always tempered ambitions, has valued privacy but most of all cherished the role of daughter, spouse and parent. Balancing these roles and yet allowing the achievement of that childhood dream of becoming a compassionate, competent physician, did not make for an easy, or a trouble-free life.

Today, I remain anguished at our inability to create a safe world for the many, but especially for the women and children exploited, kept in poverty, diseased and exposed to war, slavery, prostitution, and famine. Despite the passage of fifty years since graduation, we still have a long way to go and, unfortunately, we have to leave these efforts to our posterity.

Endnotes

1. Harvard Medical School Class of 1953, 50th *Reunion Report* 1953–2003, 198–202; 200.
2. Albert, Prof. E., *Women and the Study of Medicine,* (Vienna: Ed Alfred Holder. Hof und Universitats Buchhandler, 1895) Unpublished Trans. I.E. Low; chaps I cited.
3. Nercessian, N., *A Brief History of Women at Harvard Medical School.* Prepared for the Committee on the Celebration of Woman. (Boston: Harvard Medical School, 1995) [Chap. I. Details additional information on "The Battle for Co-Education at Harvard Medical School."]

Dr. Low was born in Italy and came to the United States in 1939. After medical school, she carried out research in virology at Harvard, followed by twenty years of research and teaching. In 1976, she undertook further training in internal medicine and infectious diseases. Subsequenty she was a hospitalist and an infectious disease consultant at the Spaulding Rehabilitation Hospital (an affiliate of the Massachusetts General Hospital). Now retired, Dr. Low continues to teach at Tufts Medical School and serves as a volunteer in free clinics. Pride in her three children and four grandchildren is a central strength in her life.

Reflections on Private and Public Health Matters: Fifteen Brief Essays

Fritz Loewenstein

The Genome

The twentieth century saw astonishing scientific advances: visualization of the outer reaches of the universe, satellite communication, computer technology, atomic and subatomic physics, genetic manipulation of plants, medical and surgical advances, and others.

Just as consequential is the definition of the human genome, which will find uses that we cannot yet foresee. Embryos used in fertilization can now be screened for genetic abnormalities, and prenatal screening can be done to detect inherited diseases. High-risk individuals can be tested for adult-onset diseases such as breast cancer, and other disorders such as Alzheimer's disease might also be detected, possibly allowing preventive treatment.

It is likely that we shall demonstrate a genetic basis for homosexuality and alcoholism, with greater tolerance and, for the latter, more effective treatment. We shall probably find genetic mutations that produce autism and other psychiatric disorders. Treatment of cancers and diabetes, which consist of different varieties, will be made more precise by discovery of their specific genetic bases. Much of this research will be done at the Broad Institute in Boston, in collaboration among Harvard, the Massachusetts Institute of Technology, and the Whitehead Institute.

The Unhealthy State of Health Care

If we assume that health care at reasonable cost is, like food and shelter, a necessity of life, the present health care system, if it can be called a system, has failed miserably. It is inefficient and far too costly.

In this wealthiest of countries over 40 million people are without health insurance and receive haphazard medical care. Those on Medicaid also receive inferior care and are not accepted by most dentists.

Many hospitals and health maintenance organizations (HMOs) are profit-making institutions. They operate under constant pressure to limit services in order to reward stockholders. In other respects, too, they incorporate some of the worst features of big business: overpaid executives, some of whom have been cited for fraud; questionable accounting practices; takeover of plans with sudden changes in costs and benefits; and closing of plans due to bankruptcy.

Between 20% and 25% of every health care dollar spent in the United States goes to administrative costs: 294 billion dollars annually! Canadian Provincial Plans spend proportionally less than one-third that amount.[1] In the Medicare Program only 6% of total money spent goes to administrative expenses.

HMOs, hospitals, and drug companies spend huge amounts of money on advertising and promotion, all of these costs ultimately borne by the consumer. Health insurance premiums, already high, have risen a further 27% for individuals during the past year, 16% for families. Small business owners can no longer afford to buy health insurance for their employees, and employees find it difficult to pay their share of the premiums. Many employers now prefer to hire part-time instead of full-time workers in order to avoid paying for health insurance. Thus more and more people are left without coverage, and middle class families are increasingly affected. It is estimated that at least 18,000 Americans aged 25 to 64 die each year due to lack of health insurance.[2] The anxieties of serious illness are compounded by worry about medical bills.

Three years ago I retired from my work as hematologist-oncologist but still do volunteer work in a free clinic for those who lack health insurance. The patients I see there are hard-working people: carpenters, roofers, cleaning ladies, taxi drivers, cooks, and so on, many earning only slightly more than minimum wage ($5.15 per hour!). Or they are unemployed, looking for work.

Local and state taxes have risen because of the increasing cost of Medicaid programs. These increases are due not only to expensive new diagnostic techniques and treatments, and to aging of the population, but also to the factors described above.

Clearly we need thorough reform of the present system. I believe that a publicly administered program of universal health insurance, similar to the Medicare program, would eliminate most of the inequities and inefficiencies. A California study showed that such a plan would cover all of the state's citizens, including the 6 million uninsured, and save over $7 billion annually in health spending. Most polls have shown that the public favors such a course.[3] Funding would need to come from payroll and income taxes, but premiums and deductibles would be small, and the overall cost to businesses and individuals would be much lower.

To achieve this will not be easy. Presidents Truman and Clinton tried and failed. The health industry has lobbies in Washington, DC, and state capitals, which influence lawmakers to prevent change. The cost of such lobbying, harmful to the consumer, is also borne by the consumer.

However, there are encouraging signs: The state of Maine is introducing a universal health plan to replace private plans. A 10,000-member organization of physicians, Physicians for a National Health Program, sponsors discussions and articles about such a plan. A recent issue of *The Journal of the American Medical Association* contains two editorials that strongly support the development of government-supervised universal health insurance.[4] In the same issue is an article by The Physicians' Working Group for a Single-Payer National Health Insurance, which gives a thorough analysis of the shortcomings of our present system. The Institute of Medicine of the National Academy of Sciences also called for a universal health care plan.[5]

There are many who disapprove of government involvement in health care. However, Medicare has been far more equitable, economic, and efficient than the profit-making health maintenance organizations, and it would be reasonable to extend the Medicare Program to cover the entire population. The savings in administrative costs alone would amount to many billions of dollars annually. None of my patients ever failed to enroll in Medicare, whereas many complained of lack of coverage, difficulty in applying for benefits, and high premiums in the private plans.

The recently enacted modification of Medicare, promoted by the Administration and narrowly passed by the Congress, takes the program in exactly the wrong direction by introducing private plans. Furthermore, the drug provisions will give high financial rewards to the pharmaceutical industry at the expense of enrolled members.

Eventually we shall adopt a nationwide single payer system supervised by the government, but for that to occur, great pressure needs to be applied on our legislators by an informed public.

Endnotes

1. Woolhandler et al., "Costs of Health Care Administration" in the US and Canada, *New England Journal of Medicine* 349 (2003), 768–775.
2. Ibid.
3. ABC NEWS – Washington Post Poll, October, 2003.
4. *JAMA,* 290 (2003), 816 and 818.
5. *New York Times* (January 15, 2004), A21.

Health Care at the End of Life

"It is as natural to die as to be born"
—Francis Bacon, Of Death (1625).

"Cowards die many times before their deaths,
the valiant never taste of death but once.
Of all the wonders that I yet have heard,
it seems to me most strange that men should fear,
seeing that death, a necessary end,

—William Shakespeare, Julius Caesar, II, ii.

Until 70 years ago people usually died at home, in familiar surroundings, and attended by family members who comforted the dying persons and quickly responded to their needs. Death now often occurs in the hospital, the patients in a cubicle filled with technical equipment, tubes running into several orifices and blood vessels. They are attended by unfamiliar faces and may be unable to make their wants known or, if they can, help does not always come. Sometimes this sort of treatment is maintained even when all hope of recovery has vanished. Patients have been kept alive artificially for years as with Karen Ann Quinlan who, at age twenty-one in 1975, became comatose and never recovered brain function. Against her family's wishes she was kept alive until 1985, with harrowing effect on her family.[1] Nancy Cruzan, at age

25 in 1983, was in an auto accident that resulted in permanent coma. A Missouri Supreme Court decision opposed removal of life support. Right to life groups intervened. Finally in 1990 a judge approved removal of the gastric feeding tube.[2]

These ordeals were publicized and led to the development of legally enforceable individual planning for end of life care. However, government interference with relatives' decisions to end life support still occurs. Florida Governor Jeb Bush, with approval of the Florida legislature, recently injected himself into such a case..

Thus it is important that everyone leave detailed directions about what measures should or should not be used in the process of dying. This health care directive is combined with the naming of a health care proxy, usually a close relative or trusted friend, in case an individual cannot make his wishes known. Permission for organ donation can be appended.

It is at this point, when a patient's life is ebbing, that the physician must fulfill one of his most important functions. I have witnessed attending physicians withdrawing from a case when life was coming to an end. Yet the physician can do much to ease the experience for the patient and his family. When the physician has become a trusted friend and advisor, his or her assurance that death will not be painful or difficult will reduce fear. And even when the patient is in throes of death, the family can be reassured that he or she is comatose and does not truly experience discomfort.

We can be inspired by a mother's account of Dr. William Osler's care of her young daughter who was dying, probably of leukemia:

> He visited our little Janet twice every day from the middle of October until her death a month later, and these visits she looked forward to with a pathetic eagerness and joy. . . . Instantly the sickroom was turned into fairyland, and in fairy language he would talk about the flowers, the birds, and the dolls. . . . In the course of this he would manage to find out all he wanted to know about the little patient.

> The most exquisite moment came one cold, raw November morning, when the end was near, and he mysteriously brought out from his inside pocket a beautiful red rose, carefully wrapped in paper, and told how he had watched this

last rose of summer growing in his garden and how the rose had called out to him as he passed by, that she wished to go along with him to see his little lassie. That evening we all had a fairy tea party, at a tiny table by the bed, Sir William talking to the rose, his "little lassie" and her mother in a most exquisite way . . . and the little girl understood that neither fairies nor people could always have the color of a red rose in their cheeks, or stay as long as they wanted to in one place, but that they nevertheless would be very happy in another home and must not let the people they left behind, particularly their parents, feel badly about it; and the little girl understood and was not unhappy.[3]

Endnotes

1. Marilyn Webb, *The Good Death* (Bantam Books, 1997) 129–153.
2. Ibid. 154–168.
3. Cushing, Harvey, *The Life of Sir William Osler,* v ii, (London: Oxford University Press, 1925) 620.

Assisted Suicide and Euthanasia

For those patients with advanced cancer and other illnesses, who are no longer responding to treatment, and who are not expected to live longer than three months, hospice programs have been developed. There they receive palliative (comfort) care. Morphine or analogous narcotics are given for pain, sometimes in insufficient doses. The physician should not hesitate to use them in fully effective amounts and should realize that, with time, doses always need to be increased. In this situation addiction is never a problem.

I have been a hematologist-oncologist and have treated many cancer patients. The nurses in our hospice program have been completely devoted to their task and have treated my patients with kindness, sympathy, and understanding. Many hospice patients can die comfortably at home rather than in the hospital.

Nevertheless, symptoms are never completely relieved. Narcotics often produce undesirable side effects, which may limit their use. Despite our best efforts, a few patients remain miserable with pain, nausea, shortness of breath, and fatigue. A common complaint is of weakness so severe that assistance is needed for the slightest tasks. Such patients will sometimes repeatedly ask that their lives be ended. The compassionate physician will not then want to prolong a suffering existence and may even decide that assisted suicide or euthanasia is justified. Euthanasia with adequate safeguards is legal in Holland and Oregon. Even where illegal, doctors have actively ended suffering patients' lives by giving large intravenous doses of barbiturates. I believe that under such extreme circumstances, and with the necessary safeguards, euthanasia will become more widely accepted. The important distinction is whether one is ending a life or an existence that can no longer be considered a life.[1]

Dr. Timothy Quill, an internist in Rochester, New York, wrote a detailed account of the case of a middle-aged woman with acute leukemia. In view of the difficulties of chemotherapy and the small chance for cure, and in agreement with her husband and son, she made the rational decision to forego treatment and to live her remaining months to the fullest at home with her family. Her overriding concern was to remain in control of her life and death. She asked Dr. Quinn to supply her with a lethal dose of a barbiturate. He did so, weighing all implications of his action. When bone pain and fever became intense, she ended her life after bidding friends, husband, and son goodbye. I was quite moved by this account and found the actions of the patient and her physician admirable.[2] Dr. Sherwin Nuland uses this case as an example of justified assisted suicide.[3]

Endnotes

1. James Rachels, *The End of Life, Euthanasia and Morality,* (London: Oxford University Press, 1986), 32–33.
2. Timothy Quinn, "Death and Dignity: A Case of Individualized Decision Making," *New England J. of Medicine* 324 (1991), 691–694.
3. Sherwin Nuland, *How We Die,* (New York: Vintage Books, 1993), 154.

Doctor and Patient

The German word for office hour is *"Sprechstunde,"* literally "speaking hour." From patients I often hear the complaint, "My doctor does not listen to me." And "He does not explain things to me." We tend to write prescriptions instead of conversing with the patient. In fact, I know psychiatrists who have almost completely stopped verbal intercourse with their patients and simply prescribe drugs. Here we can take a lesson from bartenders who know that the combination of listening and medicine (alcohol) is most beneficial.

Nurse practitioners now customarily do so-called screenings. However, it is important that the physician himself interview the patient, especially at first encounter, to learn about his life and background, to register his concerns and anxieties, and to probe for diagnostic clues. This may take between 30 and 60 minutes and should be done properly despite pressure from managers of HMOs to see a larger number of patients.

Just as important is a careful physical examination. The various scans have certainly increased our diagnostic powers, but they have not made irrelevant the physical examination. A carotid bruit, aortic or mitral murmur, palpable abdominal aortic aneurysm, and absent pulses in the feet are a few of the asymptomatic but potentially serious abnormalities that can be found. An occasional early breast cancer is palpable though not visible on mammogram. I have seen resident physicians, relying too much on scans, miss easily palpable breast and abdominal tumors. Moreover, the carefully performed physical exam reinforces the patient's perception that the doctor is truly interested in his case. During the examination the physician can also make pertinent reassuring remarks and ask further questions. Here the patient will often anxiously regard the physician's facial expression for fear that he has discovered a serious abnormality: "I observe the physician with the same diligence as he the disease."[1]

These are skills that must be emphasized and developed in our medical schools and too often are not. It is significant that the word "clinician," for one who is adept at this, has gone out of fashion.

The physician must then explain the implications of what he has found, the reason for any tests, and the purpose and possible complications of treatment. He can do much to reduce the patient's fears about unimportant symptoms or findings that have come to light. It is also good not to place too much significance on slight laboratory variations. In most laboratory testing, the limits of normal have been set arbitrarily at two standard deviations from the mean, and a few results above or below these limits are still normal.

Special skill, understanding, and empathy are required to inform a patient, especially a young or middle-aged one, that he or she has an incurable cancer. Dr. Jerome Groopman discusses this difficult task.[2]

Ideally, the patient would see the same physician on subsequent visits in order to forge a trusting and familiar relationship. Unfortunately, in the present large medical groups that is often impossible.

I would here plead for more house calls by the physician. Many ailments can be managed with a visit to those who cannot leave their homes, preventing emotionally disturbing and expensive trips to the emergency room. The physician then gains a first-hand knowledge of the patient's surroundings, his limitations, and his relations with family members.

Endnotes

1. John Donne, *Devotions upon Emergent Occasions* (1624).
2. Jerome Groopman, *The New Yorker* (October 28, 2002), 62.

Medical Education

Premedical: Incipient physicians need a broader education than they generally now receive. To be sure, a year of physics, two years of chemistry, and one or two years of biology are necessary. However, medical schools should discourage science as a major and give preference to those applicants who have majored in the humanities: the classics, languages, history, English, or philosophy. And the English would be the literature of England, rather than of America: Chaucer, Shakespeare, Milton, and the 18th and 19th century poets and novelists.1 A thorough study of the humanities will develop a mental discipline, analytical skills, an ability to reason, an understanding of human beings with their strengths and failings, and what Lewis Thomas calls, "an affection for the human condition." I quote further:

> Society would be the ultimate beneficiary. We could look forward to a generation of doctors who have learned as much as anyone can learn, in our colleges and universities, about how human beings have always lived out their lives. Over the bedrock of knowledge about our civilization, the medical schools could then construct as solid a structure of medical science as can be built, but the bedrock would always be there, holding everything else.

Medical: More emphasis needs to be placed on skillfully obtaining the history of a new patient and on performing a careful physical examination. Other facets of patient care need to be taught. (See my discussion under Doctor and Patient.) I would include a course of medical statistics, a course of ethics using as texts two books of James Rachel's, and also a course concerning the social aspects of medical care in the United States.[3, 4]

Several books would be read by all medical students, among these:

> *Migraine* by Oliver Sacks, a thorough discussion of a disorder which has been poorly understood.[5]

> *How We Die* by Sherwin Nuland, an empathic account of the ways in which life declines and ends.[6]

> *The Plague* by Albert Camus, a beautifully written novel about a bubonic plague epidemic in a French-Algerian city and its effect on various individuals.[7]

The extremely high cost of a medical education prevents many deserving students from choosing medicine as a career. A partial solution would consist of government scholarships in return for five years of practice in an underserved area.

Postgraduate: Unfortunately this has been appropriated by the pharmaceutical industry, both at university centers and at community hospitals. Educational lectures and conferences are paid for by drug companies which supply speakers and suggest topics. These almost always deal with treatment, diagnostic techniques being neglected. The newest and most expensive drugs receive most attention although they may have no advantages over older, less expensive ones. Further, new drugs have the disadvantage of not being fully evaluated. Several years are often required before harmful side effects of a drug are well understood.

A large army of detail men enters doctors' offices in order to promote their companies' products, exaggerating benefits and minimizing side effects. Doctors are bribed with free dinners, trips, and gadgets, and many then prescribe needlessly expensive drugs. The drug companies benefit; patients pay the price.

The pharmaceutical industry should be barred from taking part in medical education.[8]

Endnotes

1. Lionel Trilling, "Reflections on a Lost Cause: English Literature and American Education," in *Speaking of Literature and Society*, ed. Diana Trilling, (New York: Harcourt Brace Jovanovich, 1979) 343–360.
2. Lewis Thomas, "How to Fix the Premedical Curriculum," in *The Medusa and the Snail*, (New York: Bantam Books, 1980) 113–116.
3. James Rachels, *Can Ethics Provide Answers?* (Lanham, MD: Rowman and Littlefield, 1997).
4. Idem. *The End of Life, Euthanasia and Morality*, Oxford University Press, 1986
5. Oliver Sacks, *Migraine, Understanding a Common Disorder*, (University of California Press, 1985).
6. Sherwin Nuland, *How We Die, Reflection on Life's Final Chapter*, (New York: Vintage Books, 1995).
7. Albert Camus, *The Plague*, trans. Stuart Gilbert, (New York: The Modern Library, 1948).
8. Arnold Relman, "Doctor's Drug Problem," *New York Times*, November 18, 2003) A2.

Vitamins and Alternative Drugs

Few fields are as pervaded by misconception and falsehood as health matters. Millions of Americans take vitamin tablets needlessly. Supplementary vitamins are needed by those who suffer from malnutrition due to chronic disease, alcoholism, anorexia, or impaired intestinal absorption, but healthy people do not need to take vitamins. It takes several months for volunteers on a severely deficient diet to develop signs of B complex deficiency, and even those who subsist mainly on fast food will not develop deficiencies.

The B complex and C (water soluble) vitamins act as co-enzymes and perform their function in the most minute quantities. The Food and Nutrition Board of the National Academy of Sciences establishes recommended dietary allowances (RDAs), which are very generous and are nevertheless exceeded by almost all dietary intakes of healthy individuals.

Half of all Americans take supplementary vitamins, far in excess of RDAs. With the B complex and C vitamins these excesses are harmless, except to the pocketbook. However, the fat-soluble vitamins A and D, when taken in excess of 10,000 IU of vitamin A and 400 IU of vitamin D can produce serious toxicity. The best policy therefore is to take no supplementary vitamins unless a clear need exists.

Taking vitamin E is also unnecessary and gives no benefit. "There is little unequivocal evidence that vitamin E is of nutritional significance in human beings."[1]

Many studies have been done to establish whether vitamin E, an antioxidant, given as supplement, prevents cardiovascular disease and other disorders. None have shown such benefit. Only patients with severe intestinal malabsorption need supplementary vitamin E to prevent nerve (axonal) degeneration in the brain and spinal cord.

The use of alternative medicines should also be discouraged. The Food and Drug Administration has no control over the constituents of so-called "nature remedies." The supposedly active elements are present in widely varying amounts, thus making any beneficial effects unpredictable. Furthermore, the active ingredients occasionally produce serious harm, even death, such as the deaths caused by herbal Ephedra (ephedrine).

An excellent article in *Consumer Reports* discusses the entire problem of nature remedies and lists twelve which are hazardous.[2]

About water: It is not necessary to drink seven glasses of water daily to maintain health. Under ordinary conditions one's thirst is a good guide. Bottled water has no health advantages over municipal tap water. In fact, one study showed that 5%–10% of bottled water was contaminated with chemicals or bacteria. Municipal water supplies are monitored for contamination.

Much of the advice presented in the popular press and in advertisements about health matters is wrong or misleading. Where can the public then obtain dependable information? There are a number of sources; several are listed here with their telephone numbers:

The Harvard Health Letter and Harvard Women's Health Watch, (800-829-5921).

Mayo Clinic Health Letter, (866-516-4974).

Other medical centers, such as the Cleveland Clinic, publish similar periodicals.

The Medical Letter, (800-211-2769).

Endnotes

1. Robert Marcus and Ann Coulston in Goodman and Gilman's *The Pharmacological Basis of Therapeutics,* 10th edition, McGraw-Hill, 2001, 1786–1788.
2. "Dangerous Supplements Still at Large," *Consumer Reports,* May, 2004, 12–17.

Some Environmental Hazards

Governmental agencies have exaggerated some environmental dangers, underestimated others:?

Radon: Uranium miners have been exposed to high concentrations of radon gas and radon decay products. The latter are alpha emitters, which, when inhaled, have carcinogenic effects on the lining of the bronchial tubes. Thus they produced lung cancers in the miners.

Radon in varying concentrations is found everywhere on earth. Its concentration in homes is much lower than in mines, and many investigations have tried to determine whether domestic radon increases the incidence of lung cancer.

Most of these studies, from the United States, Canada, China and India have shown no such association. The best such study is probably one from Finland.[1] Radon concentration in Finland is unusually high, and Finns seem to live in the same home for decades. These features tend to increase the reliability of the study. Again no effect was shown on incidence of lung cancer.

Thus the warning of health departments to test for radon and to insulate basements is unnecessary.

Lead: Lead toxicity is a more serious problem than previously thought. The most severely affected are young children who ingest old lead-based paint flaking off the walls of tenement buildings or who absorb lead from the glaze of Mexican pottery. These children suffer permanent intellectual impairment. Until recently, blood levels below 10 mcg/ml were thought to be safe. However, further studies have shown that children with levels below that also have permanent mental retardation.[2] Indeed there seems to be no completely safe level.

Unfortunately, the present Administration, under pressure from the lead industry, has countermanded recommendations from involved scientists to abolish the 10 mcg/ml permissible level. We need to focus on removing children from old buildings that still contain lead paint and on educating Hispanic-American families about the hazard of lead glazed pottery.

Asbestos: Asbestos has been used as fireproofing and insulating material. Repeated inhalation of asbestos fibers causes lung fibrosis, lung cancer, and mesothelioma, a particularly virulent malignant tumor of the covering of the lung. Asbestos is still present in the walls of older public buildings such as schools and hospitals.

The concern that this asbestos is dangerous is unwarranted. As long as the material is not disturbed and dispersed into the air, it will do no harm. Therefore, attempts to remove the asbestos are misled. It is only when such buildings are demolished that workers will be exposed to danger and need to be protected?

PCBs (polychlorinated biphenyls: PCBs are electrical insulating materials. They are widely distributed environmental contaminants, are fat-soluble, and are present in high concentration in some fish in the Great Lakes. Contaminated fish consumption by mothers produced weight and activity deficits in their children.[3]

The chief concern with halogenated organic compounds in toxic spills has been cancer. In high concentrations PCBs cause cancer in animals, but no association has been found between exposure and cancers in humans.[4]

TCE (trichloroethylene): TCE is another prevalent chemical in toxic spills, having been used in dry cleaning and circuit board manufacturing. In high concentrations it causes liver cancer in mice and renal cancer in rats. In humans, kidney cancer has occurred, but only among those with very high and prolonged occupational exposure.[5]

Concentration of TCE in the air near toxic spills is much lower and such concentrations have not been shown to cause renal or other cancers.

Endnotes

1. Auvinen et al., "Indoor Radon Exposure and Risk of Lung Cancer," *Journal of the National Cancer Institute* 88 (1996) 966–402.
2. Canfield et al., "Intellectual Impairment in Children with Blood Level Concentrations below 10mcg per Deciliter," *New England J, Medicine* 348 (2003) 1517–1526.

3. Jacobson et al., "Effects of Exposure to PCBs and Related Compounds on Growth and Activity in Children," *Neurotoxicology and Teratology* 12 (1990) 319–326.
4. *Casarett and Doull's Toxicology,* ed. Klaassen, 6th edition (2001) 279.
5. Bruning and Boldt, "Renal Toxicity and Carcinogenicity of Trichloroethylene," *Critical Reviews in Toxicology* 30 (2000) 253–285.

The Pharmaceutical Industry

In large splashy advertisements the drug industry pictures itself as the most humanitarian of institutions. Ah, if it were only so! It actually is one of the more self-aggrandizing of our industries. Its products are a necessity of life, and it is the elderly who are the major consumers of medicines and who can least afford them. Nevertheless, drug company policies are designed to maximize income of stockholders and administrators at the expense of consumers.

The industry spends billions each year on advertising and promotion, more than on research and development. It has certainly developed important new drugs, sometimes at great expense, as have also the universities and the National Institutes of Health, the latter mostly through grants. However, new drugs that reach the market are often only slight modifications of existing ones, with no advantages over older, less expensive medications.

We do not need five different selective serotonin reuptake inhibitors (SSRIs), or antidepressants. "There is no good evidence that any SSRI is superior to any other for treatment of depression."[1] Similarly, we do not need nine different ACE inhibitors for treatment of hypertension. The same applies to the multiplicity of antihistamines, antibiotics, and so on.

The industry spends many millions each year to influence legislation in its favor. This was an important factor in the recent modification of the Medicare Act, which enriches drug companies at the expense of those enrolled in Medicare. All of these actions, and others, are responsible for the high cost of drugs. Proof can be seen in the great disparity in cost of brand names versus generic drugs. Will the industry police itself to stop abuses? I doubt it.

There is increasing concern that biomedical and pharmaceutical research has been influenced and motivated by financial interests. Pope John Paul II has criticized the "overriding financial interests" that operate in research fields. In his words:

> The pre-eminence of the profit motive in conducting scientific research ultimately means that science is deprived of its epistemological character, according to which its primary goal is discovery of the truth. The risk is that when research takes a utilitarian turn, its speculative dimension, which is the inner dynamic of man's intellectual journey, will be diminished or stifled.[2]

Researchers often receive grants and gifts from pharmaceutical companies or own stock in such companies. Disclosure of these connections is intended to avert criticism but does not prevent subtle bias in the scientist's work. The universities have become involved in this unholy alliance. An extreme example is the case of Dr. Nancy Olivieri who, in 1997, was dismissed by the University of Toronto after she demonstrated that a drug used to treat Mediterranean anemia and produced by Apotex Company gave no benefit but had toxic effects. The company was about to announce a $12.7 million donation to the university. Dr. Olivieri later regained her position.[3]

Hamilton Moses III of the Boston Consulting Group and Joseph Martin, Dean of Harvard Medical School, suggested a possible solution to such conflicts of interest. An organization separate from the institution and from faculty would manage stocks in companies whose products are being studied.[4]

Endnotes

1. *The Medical Letter* 45 (Nov 24, 2003), 93.
2. Pope John Paul II, in letter to the apostolic nuncio in Poland (March 25, 2002).
3. Sheldon Krimsky, *Science in the Private Interest,* Lanham MD: Rowman and Littlefield, 2003, 45–47.
4. Moses and Martin, "Academic Relationships with Industry," *Journal of the American Medical Association* 285 (2001), 933–935.

Israel and Palestine

Since 1947, when the United Nations passed the partition plan, constant conflict has existed between Arabs and Jews. This has been punctuated at times by atrocities; that is, deliberate violence against non-militants, committed by both sides. In December 1947, Arab irregulars engaged in violent attacks on Jewish civilians.[1] In April, 1948, most inhabitants of the non-belligerent Arab village of Deir Yassin were slaughtered by Jewish forces, and there were cases of rape and mutilation.[2] About 600,000 Palestinians were more or less forcibly displaced and became refugees.[3]

The massacre of hundreds of Palestinian men, women, and children in the refugee camps of Sabra and Shatila, near Beirut in 1982, has become well known. It was carried out by Christian militiamen with the passive approval of Israeli forces commanded by Ariel Sharon.

The Israeli government has made a number of huge mistakes in its relations with Arabs. The invasion and occupation of Lebanon and Beirut was a quagmire, which resulted in thousands of deaths, both civilian and military, and produced no benefit for Israel.

The second-class treatment of Israeli Arabs, forming about 20% of the population, has alienated those citizens. One suicide bomber came from this group.

The Israeli army and Israelis are hated by Palestinians as an occupying power. Every Israeli government, including that of Yitzhak Rabin, has encouraged and subsidized Jewish settlements in the West Bank and Gaza. There are now about 230,000 settlers in these enclaves, which require military protection and an intricate network of roads that are often built through Palestinian olive groves. As a result, Palestinians are blocked from traveling from one village to another. The settlements are a constant source of conflict, and no peace will be possible unless they are dismantled.

The wall recently erected to protect against suicide bombers illegally encroaches on Palestinian territory, further inciting Palestinian anger, and suicide bombers have continued to invade Israel. Deliberate intimidation and humiliation of civilians at roadblocks only increases their frustration and anger, thus fueling more suicide bombings, which should be seen as acts of desperation.

Is it right to fire into groups of stone-throwing boys? Does demolition of the homes of suicide bombers lead to peace or does it further infuriate Palestinians?

Not only are these measures wrong from a humanitarian point of view, they also work against Israel's long-term interest, for they all prevent establishment of a stable, self-sufficient Palestinian state existing alongside a secure State of Israel. Without such a Palestine, no lasting peace is possible.

The American government is partly responsible for these abuses, for it is American money that pays for Israeli arms and the military. If the U.S. government were to withhold Israel's subsidies until the dismantling of the settlements, these would disappear. We have the leverage to push events in the right direction if we would only use it!

Since biblical times morality has been an essential element of Jewish teaching: to treat others with justice, compassion, and righteousness, and to help the poor and the oppressed. These injunctions clearly extend to non-Jews:

> And a stranger shalt thou not oppress; for ye know well the spirit of the stranger, seeing ye yourselves were strangers in the land of Egypt.[4]

The prophets and Talmudic writers perpetuated these teachings. It is ironic and sad that the State of Israel, founded by Jews who themselves had suffered greatly, has largely abandoned these ideals.

Endnotes

1. Avi Shlaim, *The Iron Wall, Israel and the Arab World,* New York: Norton & Company, 2000, 27 and 83.
2. Benny Morris, *The Birth of the Palestinian Refugee Problem, 1947–1949,* Cambridge University Press, 1987, 113.
3. Idem. 298.
4. *Exodus,* XXIII, 9.

On Patriotism

Patriotism is not expressed by wrapping ourselves, our dogs, and our cars in the American flag. Rather, it consists of improving the lives of all, including those who cannot help themselves, and of fostering true democracy, even when this involves criticism of the government: "We must not confuse dissent with disloyalty."[1]

Endnote

1. Edward R. Murrow, CBS correspondent, concerning the loyalty
   hearings of Senator Joseph McCarthy, Chairman of the Subcommit-
   tee on Investigation (1954).

Our Government and Iraq

The United States government has often interfered in the affairs
of other countries. Seldom have these ventures been as misguided as the invasion of Iraq, an attack on a sovereign state,
and thus in violation of international law. The justification given
was that Iraq had developed a nuclear arms program as well as
chemical and bacterial agents, that it was allied with the Al
Qaeda network and thus partly responsible for the September
2001 attack, and that it posed an imminent threat to its neighbors
and to the United States. None of these statements were true and
were known from the beginning not to be true. The Administration deliberately ignored the reports of Hans Blix, United
Nations inspector, that Iraq had no mass weapons program. The
country and the Congress were misled into approving a military
adventure halfway around the world, an adventure extremely
costly in human lives and resources.

Thus our government involved us in an unnecessary war on
the basis of lies. A prescient passage from Heart of Darkness
comes to mind. Marlow, the protagonist says:

> You know I hate, detest, and can't bear a lie, not because I
> am straighter than the rest of us, but simply because it
> appalls me. There is a taint of death, a flavour of mortality in
> lies—which is exactly what I hate and detest in the world—
> what I want to forget. It makes me miserable and sick, like
> biting into something rotten would do.[1]

Indeed, more than two thousand American soldiers have
died, many more have been maimed and injured. The number
of Iraqi casualties is much greater, many of them civilians. Terrorism in the Middle East and elsewhere has increased. Life for
the average Iraqi has become disrupted, with street crime, lack
of social services, and random bombings. Many Iraqis, especially
Shiites, are glad to be rid of Saddam Hussein, a murderous dictator, but they resent our troops as an occupying force that has
not been able to restore tranquility.

The involvement in Iraq has already cost 90 billion dollars and will require four billion more each month. Millions are still being spent in a futile search for weapons of mass destruction, which, the Administration assures us, will be found.

Let's face it, rebuilding Iraq is going to be far more expensive than Americans have been led to believe.[2]

We need to evacuate Iraq soon and must allow the Iraqis to develop their own society and government. Civil strife may continue, but a representative government is likely to emerge. Its resources, including oil, must be in Iraqi, not American, hands.

Endnotes

1. Joseph Conrad, *Heart of Darkness,* New York: Harper & Brothers, 1910.
2. Donald Hepburn, "Nice War. Here's the Bill," *New York Times,* September 3, 2003, Op-Ed page.

National Policies

Our government is spending many billions of dollars on ventures that are of benefit to the defense and space industries but not to the country. We maintain a huge military machine, which is not necessary to combat terrorism. One billion dollars are being spent to dispose of sarin nerve gas. But what madness to produce that stuff in the first place!

Astronomers and physicists agree that the manned space program has no scientific value. Two crews have perished. Yet the Administration plans to continue and expand the program at great cost. The Hubble telescope, on the other hand, consuming only a small part of NASA's budget, has greatly increased our knowledge of the universe. Ironically, funding for this unmanned telescope is being reduced, so that it will stop functioning by 2007.[1]

Much money is wasted by awarding contracts without competitive bidding to large companies like Halliburton. Many millions are consumed in unnecessary subsidies for agribusiness, the sugar industry, tobacco farming, and pork projects.

Present tax policies favor large corporations, many of which move headquarters offshore to escape taxes altogether. American companies defer paying taxes on foreign profits if the money is kept outside the United States. Billions in taxes are lost thereby.[2] This is another instance of the inordinate influence large corporations have on federal policy.

The tax cut enacted two years ago, meant to stimulate the economy, has not done so, and has been of benefit only to the upper five percent of income earners. Did we not learn in the Reagan years that "trickle down economics" does not work?

Abolition of taxes on dividends and of the inheritance tax again benefits only the wealthy at the ultimate expense of those with modest means.

Federal spending is out of control, with a $500 billion deficit this fiscal year. Again, who benefits from this huge debt? It is those who lend money. The average taxpayer will bear the ultimate burden of paying off the debt and its interest.

The undesirable effects of all these political actions are mainly two: They increase the already great disparity between the wealthy and the poor. Second, profligate federal spending diverts resources from domestic needs, which are increasingly neglected. Recently all branch libraries in my home city were closed because of lack of funds. Many of the users were schoolchildren who were unable to travel to the central library. We need to ask ourselves: What is more important in maintaining a healthy democracy, a well-read public or an imperial military machine?

Many other domestic programs are being reduced or cut because of lack of funds. Funding for education is reduced, including the care of children with disabilities. Supervision of national and state parks suffers because the number of rangers is being decreased. Other instances could be listed. All this at a time when billions are being wasted by the federal government.

Endnotes

1. Michael Benson, *New York Times,* January 31, 2004) A17.
2. *New York Times,* October 2, 2003, A1.

Poverty

There is a great underclass of citizens who live in extreme poverty and who have no political voice. Their number increases because the number of unemployed and underemployed has grown.[1] To our shame be it said: the legal minimum wage is still $5.15 per hour with no prospect of an increase, many workers earning only \$6.50 or \$7 hourly, while legislators and government employees receive regular raises. Many people need to hold two jobs to remain afloat. The Administration's claim that our economy is healthy is probably based on stock market performance and does not acknowledge that jobs are disappearing.

In some areas the unemployment rate is much higher than the national average of 6%–7%. In our inner cities more than half of black men are unemployed, many of them then attracted to drug trafficking and other crimes. Other social ills follow.

Several suggestions: A federal program similar to the Civil Conservation Corps (CCC) of the 1930s could be instituted, to give useful work to unemployed young men and women. These would repair and construct public buildings, patrol natural refuges, protect and maintain parks, and so on. Young children in the inner cities could receive daily care in municipal preschool classes. Schools would improve in funding and quality so as to match those in the suburbs. Children must be removed from violent or turmoil filled homes. Neighborhood clinics need to be established.

Endnote

1. Paul Krugman, "Jobs, Jobs, Jobs," *New York Times,* February 10, 2004

War

Wars are the ultimate public health disaster. Modern wars inevitably kill and injure more civilians than militants. Massacres of non-combatants have become common.

Large populations are deprived of food, water, and shelter and become refugees. Poor sanitation and malnutrition lead to epidemics, and medical supplies and personnel are often absent.

Land mines are the terrible aftermath of war. Hundreds of children are killed and maimed every year by mines. It should be known that our government refused to sign the international treaty to outlaw land mines.

The invasion of Iraq was a serious mistake, and we also should not meddle in Haiti's affairs. But what should be done about countries such as Yugoslavia, Iraq, and the Sudan, ruled by dictators who torture and slaughter their citizens? It is not the United States that should try to set this right, rather it should be the United Nations or a regional organization such as NATO or the Organization of African States.

Four anti-war novels I recommend:

All Quiet on the Western Front by Erich Maria Remarque (1925), a beautifully written, graphic, affecting account of the life of a German soldier on the Western Front in World

Johnny Got His Gun by Dalton Trumbo (1939), the fictional account of a young American soldier rendered quadriplegic and mute in World War I.

Catch 22 by Joseph Heller (1955), a seriocomic, satiric description of life in an Air Force unit in North Africa and Italy during World War II.

The Naked and the Dead by Norman Mailer (1948), an epic novel depicting the physical and emotional degradation of jungle warfare on a Pacific island in World War II.

Passages in *Gulliver's Travels,* especially in "A Voyage to the Houyhnhnms," criticize war. "The Trade of a Soldier is held the most honorable of all others: Because a Soldier is a Yahoo hired to kill in cold Blood as many of his own Species, who have never offended him, as possibly he can."[1]

Falstaff, the realist, answers Prince Hal, warrior-prince: "Can honor set to a leg? No. Or an arm? No. Or take away the grief of a wound? No. —"[2]

In short, there have always been those who decried the senselessness of war. Despite Machiavelli, Kissinger, and Bush, the true Realpolitik is: violence breeds violence.

Endnotes

1. Jonathan Swift, *Gulliver's Travels* (1726).
2. William Shakespeare, *Henry IV,* Part I, Act V, Sc 1, 131.

Guns

Another public health problem: I am astonished and mystified by the American obsession with guns. Over 7000 people were murdered with handguns in 2002.[1] A truly civilized society would not permit the prevalence of such weapons. That is to say, we need much more stringent gun control.

Endnote

1. *New York Times,* February 24, 2004, A25.

Dr. Loewenstein practiced hematology and oncology for forty-five years in Binghamton, New York, and for twenty-five years he was associated with the Oncology Clinic at Syracuse University Medical School. During that time he participated in several clinical research projects, two of which were published. He is presently retired but continues to do volunteer work in a primary care clinic for patients without health insurance. He plays violin in the Tri-Cities Opera orchestra, and plays both violin and viola for pleasure and in performances.

Address to Be Given on Receipt of the Plessner Prize

Wendy Ring

When the members of the Harvard Medical School class of 1953 were asked to submit essays, Henry Ring wrote that, because of the recent death of his wife, he felt unable to contribute. He proposed instead that we substitute an address that his daughter Wendy had written. The occasion for the address was the award ceremony for a prize to be awarded to her by the California Medical Association. Henry wrote, by way of background:

> *For about 15 years, Wendy has had a mobile medical office in sparsely populated rural northern California. She goes to rural communities that are without adequate health care facilities to provide care for the homeless, the mentally ill, the elderly, for high school students, and for patients with substance abuse problems. Wendy started alone, with a pick-up truck and a trailer. Her organization now consists of eighteen people operating out of large vans. Her Mobile Medical Office is organized as a not-for-profit corporation funded by grants from local organizations, the state and the federal government.*

> *In 2003, Wendy was one of four recipients of the Pride in the Profession Award. She also received the Plessner Award, which is given annually by the California Medical Association to the state's outstanding rural physician. She was to receive the award at the annual meeting of the California Medical Association, but was unable to attend the meeting because she returned home to be with her mother, then dying from cancer.*

> *Even though Wendy is not a Harvard Medical School graduate, this is such an inspiring story that we decided to include*

it. She is, after all—thanks to her father's influence—an indirect product of the school. Her address, as she planned to give it, follows. —Editors.

~

In the old days, the obligations of a village healer were simple: to care for the people of your village and to train someone to take over when you are old and can no longer provide care yourself. Today I am struggling to understand my obligations as a healer in a global village where violence is epidemic, infections travel on airplanes, radioactive fallout flies on the wind and children in one country die of malnutrition, infection and trauma due to the economic policies of another. In a global village, death respects no borders, and all the smallpox vaccine and duct tape in the world can't keep us from experiencing the consequences of our actions. As doctors, we know this better than most people, and we must speak out and teach as if the survival of the species and the planet depended on it.

In the face of all this, it is easy to feel helpless. What I thought I would do now, instead of depressing you further, is to cheer you up by telling you some success stories from my practice. The first story I'd like to tell you is about how my clinic got started. I live in a rural county, which is about a six hour drive up a winding two-lane highway north of San Francisco and has an average population density of 35 people per square mile. Back in 1990 when I started my clinic, our county had a severe lack of health services for low-income people.

The mobile clinic idea came to me one day, and I just couldn't get it out of my head. Having previously been the medical director of two small community clinics, I was not naïve about what was involved. I knew I could never do it alone. But I wondered . . . if I offered to go to these underserved areas and provide the medical care, would the communities want the service enough to provide the resources to make it work? So I bought an old truck and a 24 foot travel trailer, filled a room in my house with medical supplies, and offered my services as a kind of spiritual experiment, or perhaps you could call it a medical stone soup, to see if one person's intention could bring about something larger than herself.

The result of that experiment is an established community clinic on wheels with a staff of eighteen, including two doctors, a nurse practitioner, three counselors, two case managers and two mobile units that provide services to a homeless shelter, a food bank, two soup kitchens, high risk teens at two public high schools and three small towns without physicians. Let me tell you about some of our patients.

Last year a social worker from another community agency told our administrator a story. Ten years ago when she was addicted to drugs, prostituting herself for money, and on the verge of losing custody of her children, she came to our clinic. That single encounter in which she was touched and treated with respect reawakened her to her own value and humanity and inspired her to change her life and ultimately return to work with people who are like her former self.

Another young woman first came to the clinic in early recovery from methamphetamine addiction. At our first encounter, I was struck by two things: her joyous demeanor and her early hypertensive nephropathy. She had never in her life had an ongoing relationship with a primary care physician and didn't trust doctors because of past encounters where she felt treated like a second-class citizen because she was black, female, and poor. Titration of her blood pressure medications brought her to the clinic every two weeks where I was able to note her pressured speech, absence of social connections, and a life repeatedly derailed by impulsive bad decisions. After some discussion, we started her on mood leveling medication. Today she is the manager of a halfway house and, after four successful semesters of community college, is transferring to a California State University. She is an outspoken advocate for poor women and an asset to the community.

A former needle exchange patient of ours came by recently to thank us. He has been off drugs six months and is employed at a job he loves. He said we "planted a spark in his heart" that helped him get off heroin. Another former patient stopped by to tell us that he's been sober for several years and is now a minister who is helping others.

Last year a teen-age girl at one of our local high schools came in asking to be tested for sexually transmitted infections. She had been drinking heavily at a party and woke up the next morning naked with a young man she didn't remember. Further discussion revealed that she was drinking to the point of blackout almost every weekend and smoking marijuana daily. She

269

had no coping mechanisms for stress and no ideas about fun that didn't involve substance abuse. I did an exam and some lab work, started her on contraception, and referred her to a counselor. When I saw her in follow-up a few months later, she was another person, vibrant and full of energy and enthusiasm. She had a job, was applying to college, and was involved in a peer outreach program. I don't think she had any idea of the kind of future she had narrowly averted.

I particularly remember another patient who first came to the clinic with a prescription he couldn't afford to fill. He was dirty and ragged from sleeping in the bushes. He told me that he had worked with his hands all his life but had to quit working because he developed painful non-healing sores on his hands following any minor trauma. He had been to the emergency room and the community clinic several times, each time receiving a prescription for antibiotics, which did nothing to alleviate his condition. I pulled a dermatology book off the shelf in the mobile clinic and diagnosed my first case of porphyria cutana tarda. I referred him to an internist who arranged with the blood bank for phlebotomy. The last time I saw him he was clean and well dressed and had come back not for medical care but to tell me that he was housed and back at work. He said, "Thank you for giving me back my life."

I know these stories sound like Prozac ads, and you're probably wondering when I'm going to start talking about Jesus and asking for contributions. I'm not. I just want to say that when we assure people that their lives are valuable, they respond by valuing their lives and the lives of other people. If we treat people as if their lives have no worth, it is not surprising that they end up believing that all human life is cheap. Sometimes this seems like a huge undertaking beyond what any of us can muster, but surprisingly often all it takes is the willingness to see past the problems and differences to the essential humanity of another person. I have learned from my patients that even when the problems seem insurmountable, one person following his or her heart can make a great deal of difference in the world. If we all did it, what a different world this would be!

Dr. Henry Ring, an ophthalmologist at the University of Miami, offers the following biographical information about his daughter:

"Wendy received her undergraduate degree from Yale and her M.D. and Public Health degrees from Columbia. She is an activist working to protect the environment and advocate of a single payer health care system. She is married and her son, Joshua, is a senior in high school. Her interests include hiking, backpacking, bicycling, gardening and caring for her animals, which include goats, chickens, ducks, a rabbit and a dog."